CHECK UP from the NECK UP
Ensuring your mental health in the new millennium

Joan Andrews, MFCC   Denise E. Davis, MFCC

Check Up from the Neck Up:
ensuring your mental health in the new millennium
by
Joan Andrews and Denise Davis

Published by: **Hope Press** P.O. Box 188, Duarte, CA 91009 U.S.A.
For other books by Hope Press see insert card in the back.
No parts of this book may be reproduced or transmitted in any form or by any means, electronic or mechanical, including photocopying or recording or by any information storage and retrieval system without written permission form the authors, expect for the inclusion of brief cited quotations in a review or article.
Copyright © 1999 by Joan Andrews and Denise Davis

Library of Congress Cataloging-in-Publication Data

Andrews, Joan, 1939-
  Check up form the neck up: ensuring your mental health in the new millennium/Joan Andrews, Denise E. Davis
  p. cm.
 Includes bibliographical references and index
 ISBN 1-878267-09-4
  1. Mental health--Popular works. 2. Anxiety--Popular works. 3. Depression Mental--Popular works. 4. Psychiatry--Popular works. I. Davis, Denise E. (Denise Evelyn), 1957- II. Title

RA790 .A63 2000
616.89--dc21

00-036948

CHECK UP from the NECK UP
Ensuring your mental health in the new millennium

Joan Andrews, MFCC   **Denise E. Davis, MFCC**

Joan's Acknowledgements

To the next generation; my grandchildren
  Max, Mario, Zachary, Nathan,
  and those yet to come.

Denise's Acknowledgements

In loving memory of my father, Robert Dean Davis,
  Whose zest and love for life never faltered.
To all of my clients and friends
  who shared their stories through laughter,
  tears, and triumphs.

Table of Contents

Foreword iv
Introduction
Check Up From The Neck Up 1
Chapter 1
Overwhelm 23
Chapter 2
Stress Reduction 33
Chapter 3
Problem-Solving 43
Chapter 4
Organization 57
Chapter 5
Time Management 69
Chapter 6
Procrastination 89
Chapter 7
Clutter 99

Table of Contents

Chapter 8
Consistency 113
Chapter 9
Impulsivity 121
Chapter 10
Distractibility 133
Chapter 11
Strategies for Death,
Taxes and Other
Necessary Evils 143
Chapter 12
Money 167
Chapter 13
Self-Sabotage 177
Chapter 14
Late Again 191

Chapter 15
Foot-In-Mouth Syndrome 203
Chapter 16
Moods 213
Chapter 17
Depression 227
Chapter 18
Shame and Guilt 245
Chapter 19
Anger 257
Chapter 20
Grief 269
Chapter 21
Help For Yourself In A Relationship 279
Chapter 22
Help For Your Partner and Family 289

Table Of Contents

Chapter 23
Intimacy 307
Chapter 24
Sex 329
Chapter 25
Problems at Work 349
Chapter 26
Problems With Parenting 365
Chapter 27
Problems At School 387
Chapter 28
Balance In Life 413
Chapter 29
Diet 423
Chapter 30
Exercise 433

Chapter 31
Sleep 439

Chapter 32
Hyperactivity vs. Hypoactivity 455

Chapter 33
Addictions 465

Chapter 34
Spirituality 487

Chapter 35
Co-Occurring Conditions 501

Chapter 36
Menopause 515

Foreword

Most of us have the good fortune to be born with all the right genes such that our brains work well. Temporary adversities may produce a few bad days, but in general we respond well to stress and life in general. Unfortunately, there are a very sizeable number of us who are born with a less than perfect set of genes and as a result we have some imbalances in our brain chemistry. The resulting effect on our lives can be a minor inconvenience or more severe, causing constant and irritating difficulties, or these changes can cause a major, daily disruption in our lives. Most people experience a continuum of symptoms of depression, mood swings, anxiety, phobias, irritability, anger, rage, or difficulties with paying attention, motivation, organization or chronic fatigue. Those with the most extreme problems may need medications to correct these changes in brain chemistry. However, those with less extreme problems may simply need some advice on better ways to organize, run, and manage their lives. This book, *Check Up from the Neck Up*, a check up for the brain, is designed to help this vast group of individuals who could function much better if they had some guidelines on how to cope with a brain that doesn't work quite right. Joan Andrews and Denise Davis have had years of experience counseling adults with Attention Deficit Disorder, substance abuse, depression and other problems arising from a dysfunctional brain and they now pass some of these experiences on to you. If you even opened the cover of this book, you are likely to benefit from their sage advice.

David E. Comings, M.D.
Director, Tourette Syndrome and ADHD Clinic
City of Hope National Medical Center
Duarte, CA

Check Up from the Neck Up

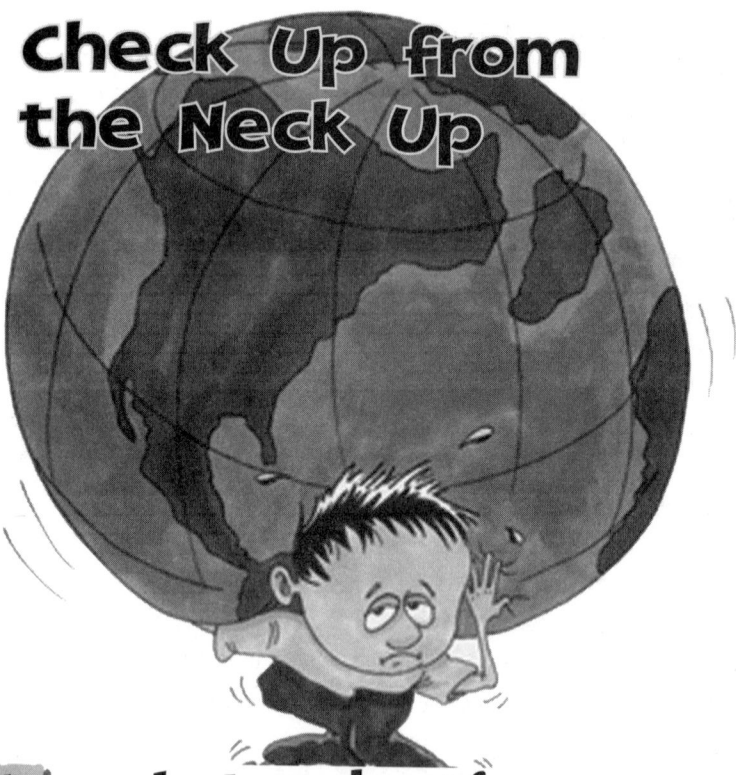

Introduction

What You Need To Know

Check Up From the Neck Up is a quick resource guide for adults who have certain difficulties operating in the world due to obsessions, compulsions, ADD, depression/moodiness, rage attacks, or other troublesome conditions. It is not a textbook. It is not meant to be read and ingested in one or several sittings. Instead, it is meant to be kept in your briefcase, on your desk, or in your nightstand for quick reference when you hit a problem area.

Each of the authors is an AESOP. Our descriptions and solutions come from direct personal experience as well as from numerous ideas and suggestions our clients have shared. We've both struggled with our special operating problems and celebrated when we've come across a tool or technique that works. We hope this book makes it easy to find and use tools that have an immediate, positive impact on your lives.

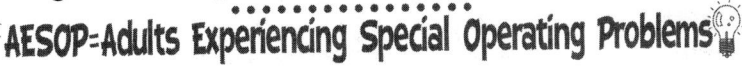

AESOP=Adults Experiencing Special Operating Problems

Who Should Read this Book?

Let's face it! There are very few of us who can be considered "perfectly normal," without any quirks or flaws. In fact, most of us have bits and pieces of certain symptoms. If you've picked up this book, chances are you may be struggling with some of these bits and pieces and are looking for solutions. You may have a little bit of depression that makes it hard to get up in the morning. Perhaps you have a little bit of anxiety and really hate walking into a room filled with strangers. You may have trouble starting (or completing) a weekly expense report. As these quirks are typically not sufficiently severe to keep us from handling a job, maintaining a relationship, or finding some joy in life, we usually just live with them.

> *"Very few of us can be considered "perfectly normal," without any quirks or flaws."* -Joan and Denise

In past years, psychologists and psychiatrists

have attributed this level of quirkiness to patterns present in families. If we are slightly depressed, they have credited it to a family system where the mother or father was depressed and passed that behavior pattern on to the next generation. With advances in science, we are gaining a new understanding of the role that brain chemistry plays in many of our quirks. We are now realizing that a great deal of who we are is made up by our genes. Our genetic makeup determines how our brains send and receive certain chemicals. The complicated action of the brain using these chemicals predisposes us toward certain emotional responses and behaviors. Thus at birth, an infant may come into the world with a predisposition toward depression due to their genetic makeup. Of course, the final layering on top of the mix is the home environment which can certainly either soften the effect of a genetic trait or make it much more pronounced.

Understanding that brain chemistry and

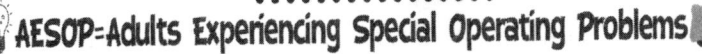

genetics play an important part in an AESOP's life will help you use some of the upcoming techniques more effectively.

What Is an AESOP?

AESOP stands for Adults Experiencing Special Operating Problems.

We decided that this book would be more helpful if we grouped the types of problems you might experience into a term we could use throughout the book. In a nutshell, we are talking about adults who for some reason or another are experiencing "special operating problems." As we played with words to find an acronym, we came up with AESOP, Adults Experiencing Special Operating Problems. The connection fits. Remember Aesop's Fables? They are short stories about animals representing everyday events and characters with whom you can easily identify. Usually, one of the characters has some type of trouble operating in the world. The hare in the "The Tortoise and the Hare" does everything very fast, yet has no consistency of performance. The boy in, "The Boy Who Cried Wolf" (formally known as "The Shepherd Boy and the Wolf") lied time after time to either get attention or simply provide some excitement in his life. These traits get them both into trouble. The moral in each story is specific to that fable, however, the overall thread is that we need to learn from our mistakes and develop new ways of operating. *Check Up From The Neck Up* is chock-full of new ways of operating.

> "...we need to learn from our mistakes and develop a new way of operating."
> -Joan and Denise

Note: The acronym "AESOP" may alternate with "Adults with SOP" throughout the book.

How to Use this Book

In each chapter you will find five main sections:

What You Need To Know

This section is meant to outline the problems that many AESOPs

 AESOP=Adults Experiencing Special Operating Problems

have with a specific topic.

and HOW TO's. You will have plenty of things to try.

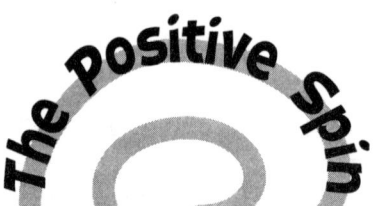

The Positive Spin

We all get into ruts. This section is meant to shake you loose so that you can conceptualize your particular problem in a different way--so that you can see your problems in a different light.

Techniques

Now to the nitty-gritty. Each chapter has SPECIFIC IDEAS

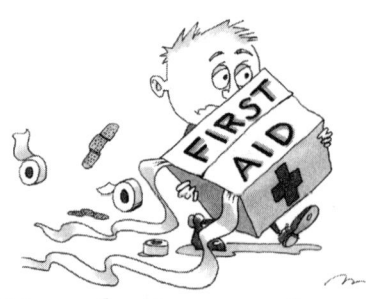

Need More First Aid?

This provides a cross-reference to other chapters that

will give more tools and shed additional light on how to tackle a problem area.

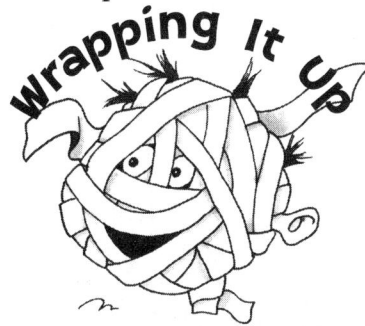
Wrapping It Up

The final section provides a summary of the most important points in the chapter. Once you have read the chapter, you can quickly flip to the summary for a review. You can even begin with the summary (how many of us flip to the end of a chapter first?) to decide if the chapter will be relevant to your needs.

Special Tips to Our Readers

KEEP MOVING, KEEP PUSHING ON, KEEP LOOKING:

If the first sentence or two in a chapter doesn't grab you, try another chapter. It may be that in your mind you've always thought that you had problems with organization, but you really have problems with procrastination. Be creative. Read the quotations from random chapters to see if they apply to you. You may find connections that we never saw and be able to construct your own unique coping tools.

What if the Techniques Don't Work?

If one technique doesn't work, try another one. Use part of one and part of another. Add your own ideas.

Use the Internet

In writing this book, it was our intention to provide websites that would expand your information on AESOPs and give you resources. What we discovered is that websites come and go without much warning. So we have decided to give you general web search ideas instead. Try using key words such as "depression," "Attention Deficit Disorder," or "Obsessive-Compulsive Disorder" to search the web for ways to expand your knowledge and resources.

Stay Positive

Remember that the positive aspects of AESOPs include

creativity, enthusiasm, and having fun with life. Check your thinking! It is easy to get mired in the idiosyncrasies and glitches that are present in the stereotypes of Adults with SOP, and to forget all the fun.

Common AESOP Traits

Even though each AESOP is an individual, we do share several common traits.

Impulsivity

Many Adults with SOP are impulsive in thoughts, speech, and action. We may blurt out hurtful or inappropriate comments before we think of the consequences. We may make many school, job, or relationship changes on a whim, again without thinking of the consequences.

Learning Problems

About 40% of the AESOP population have problems

> "Remember that the positive aspects of AESOPs include creativity, enthusiasm, and having fun with life."
> *-Joan and Denise*

AESOP=Adults Experiencing Special Operating Problems

in school. Often we have problems understanding what we read or are very slow readers. Problems with math, or with writing reports, essays or even letters, are also common for Adults with SOP. We may have great ideas and be able to talk anyone's arm off, but when it comes to writing anything down on paper our effort may look more like that of a much younger person.

Depression:

Many AESOPs have low levels of depression that, in many cases, have been present since childhood. Because it has been with us all of our lives, we may not recognize it as depression and may even be emphatic that we are not depressed. Yet, if the question is put to us in a different way, the depression often becomes evident. As Adults with SOP we can ask ourselves if we feel that the world is somehow flat, without peaks of happiness or joy, or gray instead of bright and sparkling. We may identify with these descriptions and be amazed that this state of being is called "depression."

Moods and/or Rage

Ups and downs triggered by chance comments from co-workers or partners are part of many AESOPs' worlds. Starting the day feeling OK and then plunging into the depths of despair for no obvious reason can also be a daily occurrence. Not being able to shake a mood, even when you don't want to be moody, can also be a daily occurrence.

Disorganization

Often the AESOP is surrounded by stacks of papers or a general clutter. We may claim that, though our desk or work space looks cluttered, we know where everything is located. We are sure that we can put our hands on a needed piece of paper. (When we're realistic, we may admit this is generally not true.)

Trouble Starting or Finishing Projects

Some of us procrastinate

when faced with a new project. We overwhelm ourselves and manage to do several other little things rather than getting started on the bigger one. Some of us can get started on a project with gung-ho enthusiasm and then just lose steam as the project drags on--in fact, it drags on so very long that we'd rather get started on something new and fresh rather than completing the old task.

Addictions

Adults with SOP are forever attempting to correct an inconsistent body chemistry. We may find that the caffeine in coffee or Mountain Dew perks us up and allows us to function. We may find that alcohol or marijuana calms us down, and without it, we can't sit still or can't fall asleep at night or calm our thoughts. Obviously, using substances over time sets the AESOP population up for addictions. Along with addiction to the use of these substances, we find food, sexual, and even electronic addictions as well.

Introduction • Check Up from the Neck Up

> "When we think of kids with SOP, we often think of a kid in a classroom or on the playground who is going 100 miles an hour and simply can't sit still."
> -Joan and Denise

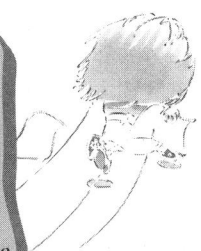

Hyperactivity

When we think of kids with SOP, we often think of a kid in a classroom or on the playground who is going 100 miles an hour and simply can't sit still. We Adults with SOP often don't look that hyperactive on the outside as we have learned to mask our hyperactivity to blend in with society. If, however, you ask us how we are feeling INSIDE, we may often admit that we are going 100 miles an hour, too.

Hypoactivity

This category describes the opposite end of the continuum. AESOPs who are hypoactive are often not identified. Instead, we get the bad rap of being lazy or unmotivated. We are accused of never doing anything in life when, in fact, because of our SOP, we may not be able to get our own systems jump-started.

Rage Attacks

Sometimes AESOPs may be easily provoked to aggression, anger, or even rage attacks. Often this rage appears without warning and may be a sign of over-arousal of our nervous systems.

Particular Pitfalls for AESOPs and Strategies to Cope with Them

Adults with special operating problems often hesitate to even try to use a self-help book. Why? Because we may have felt like total failures in the past. We may be reluctant to subject ourselves to even one more attempt at solving problems in our lives.

Coping with Failure

Often we AESOPs feel like describing ourselves as total failures in life. We may have trouble starting things, or finishing things. We may have good intentions, but terrible follow through. We can't be consistent. We blurt out an opinion or an unkind remark when we should keep quiet.

AESOPs need to understand what we perceive to be failures in a different way. This overhauled perception will provide us with a fresh outlook and some alternative routes to getting ahead in life.

Many of the feelings of failure, the feelings of being blocked, of not accomplishing something, have to do with behaviors and behaviors only. Some of these feelings are triggered by brain chemistry and may not be an accurate reflection of what is happening in our real world. Behaviors and brain chemistry can be managed, and that is what this book is all about.

On the positive side, what sets Adults with SOP apart is our creativity. We may have the ability to envision what is possible and generate not just one, but a multitude of ideas for solutions. When it comes to ourselves, this may be our hardest task; to see a vision of what should or could be different in our lives if we viewed our traits with more positive eyes. Realize that the step-by-step process of following through with new behaviors can accomplish major changes in how you see yourself and how you operate more effectively in your world.

> *"First of all, understand that as an Adult with SOP you will never be consistent with anything."*
> -Joan and Denise

Strategies for Keeping on Track

Adults with SOP often have absolutely fantastic ideas. Many of our great innovators, such as Thomas Edison and Walt Disney, are identified as being AESOPs. Our AESOP frustration often comes from not being able to follow our inspiration all the way to a conclusion.

Look at it this way: Adults with SOP, with our creativity,

have the ability to approach problems in life in many different ways. For us, there is not just one path, but six different paths (some straight, some circular) all leading to the same end. One path may take ten minutes to navigate. One path (our circular path) may take two days. One path may have a grassy patch perfect for a nap. We Adults with SOP on our path may not reach our goal for two or three days or even longer. The goals may change along the way to an even more promising path. This book will give you tips that will allow you to reach your goals.

Strategies for Being Consistent

First of all, understand that as an Adult with SOP you will never be consistent with anything. It is simply not in your nature.

Change your viewpoint. Don't even strive for absolute consistency. Does this mean you'll never finish anything? No, it means that you need to take a different mental approach to be successful as well as to feel successful.

Instead of thinking "I must be consistent," think "I must get started." Next, check on how your system or your project is going. This is the evaluation phase. Then, focus on keeping the momentum going for a while. Learn not to panic when you inevitably find yourself at a dead stop, possibly because you are bored or feel your attention being tugged in another direction. Most importantly, don't think of this as failure.

Working in peak periods interspersed with periods of down time is a normal AESOP pattern. This pattern is not a failure on your part. It is not a character flaw. It is part and parcel of our AESOP biochemical pattern, and it can be successfully managed.

Strategies when Feeling Overwhelmed

Faced with a stack of bills to pay, a report to write, a room to paint, or a garden to plant, we AESOPs often feel overwhelmed. This feeling of being overwhelmed has nothing to do with our actual ability to do the task. Instead, it has to do with the mental or physical energy required to jump in and BEGIN the task. When the feeling of being overwhelmed hits, the brakes slam on and we usually find ourselves at a dead halt.

Once we begin to feel overwhelmed, typically, the feelings of guilt ("Why can't I get started on this, what is wrong with me?") or despair ("I'll never be able to get this done") can set in. This compounds the problem and we find ourselves

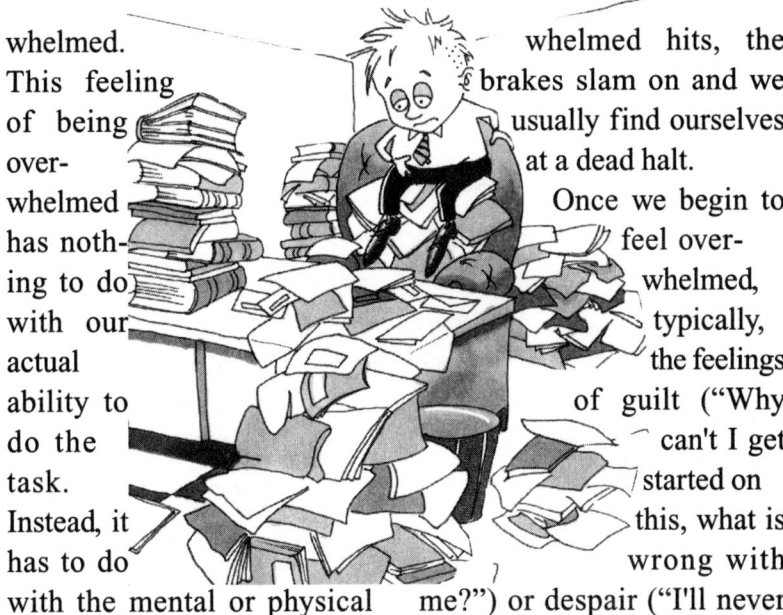

even more firmly mired in hardening cement.

Again, we must learn not to panic! For AESOPs, even when we're reading a self-help book, feeling overwhelmed is normal. The important thing is to step back, take a deep breath and remember that we are looking for specific strategies to help us change certain behaviors or feelings.

Keep Moving, Stay Positive
We encourage you to make this book your own. Mark in it, turn pages down, highlight what works, cross out what doesn't work. This is a workbook, a play book, and a solution book. Read on...

AESOP=Adults Experiencing Special Operating Problems

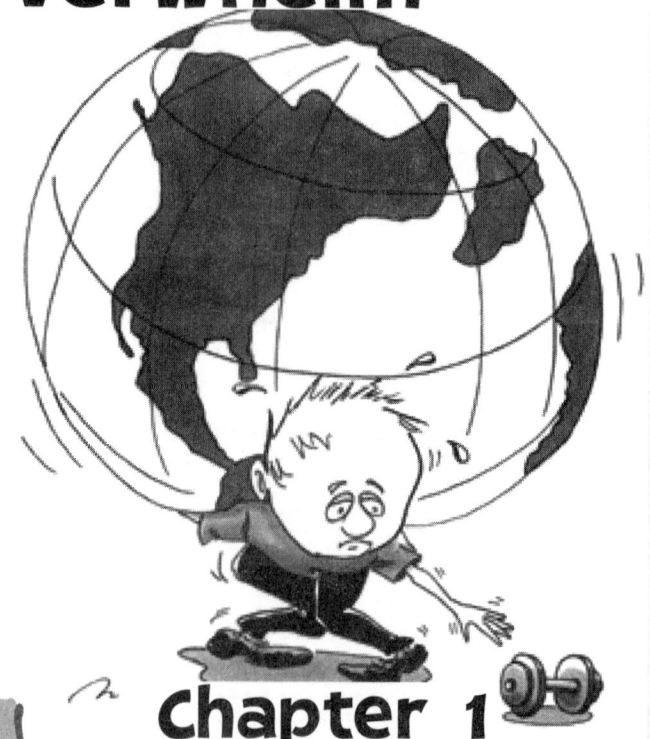

What You Need To Know

You have a list that never ends. You sometimes sit on the couch or at your desk in the middle of the day and can't figure out what to do next. You're feeling overwhelmed.

The AESOP mind can often be tremendously creative, full of ideas, quick to move off on tangents and often overcrowded. This produces a feeling of being overwhelmed and often causes the AESOP brain to feel like it has come to a dead halt or is incapable of fitting into "normal" everyday functions.

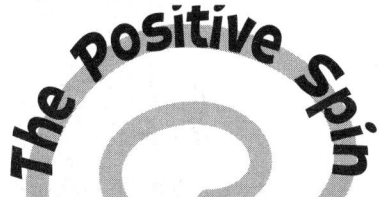

The Positive Spin

When you feel overwhelmed and are at a standstill, don't think of it as failure. Instead, recognize this phenomenon as a very normal pattern. For AESOPs, it isn't the fact that the task is too difficult or beyond our reach; instead, it is an inability to muster up enough mental or physical

AESOP=Adults Experiencing Special Operating Problems

energy to begin the task, or to continue with it once we have been sidetracked, often by some other "important" idea.

Another reality is that an AESOP's list never ends. Due to our creativity and imagination, there is always one more job, one more idea, one more book to write. This feeling of the list being unending also contributes to a sense of being overwhelmed. Surrender to the fact that you'll never get it all done. In fact, horror of horrors, if your list were all done, you would find yourself with nothing to do--another AESOP nightmare!

Techniques
Self-Awareness Strategies
Ask yourself:

Are there elements of depression present? Severe depression, which sends you under your covers for days

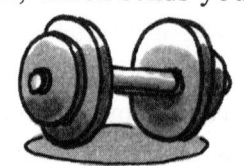

Chapter 1 • Overwhelm

> "Any idiot can face a crisis--it's the day to day living that wears you out."
> -*Anton Chekhov*

at a time, is easy to recognize. However, for the AESOP depression is more likely to be low level and insidious, thus less easily recognized. If the world seems flat or gray and life holds no spark, investigate whether an element of depression is causing you to feel overwhelmed.

Become aware of your own cyclical patterns:

If you find yourself feeling overwhelmed at certain periods of time, such as in the Fall or during the holidays, be aware of this. If you typically come to a dead halt as the days shorten and the weather changes, you might be dealing with an undiagnosed case of SAD, Seasonal Affective Disorder. If the holidays bring you to a grinding halt, you might need to look at interactions within the family and identify why this is such a difficult time. Approaching your individual patterns in this manner gives you something specific to work with rather than leaving you with a global feeling of being overwhelmed and at a loss.

Are you a "Yes" person?

Is it impossible for you to say "No" to anyone asking for a favor? Are you the first person to volunteer to help move your co-worker in the 35-foot moving van? Are you the neighbor who dog sits, cat sits, or plant sits for most of the neighborhood? Do you typically have neighborhood children in addition to your own in your house daily? Always saying yes may be the factor that is overloading you. A good book on how to say no, a conversation with a friend who will support your efforts to say no, or some professional help may be the ticket for you.

Specific Tools

Use systems:

Even though establishing a routine can be hard, devising your own system to tackle overwhelming feelings or sit-

> "I try to take one day at a time, but sometimes several days attack me at once."
> -Ashleigh Brilliant

uations brings some order to the chaos. As an Adult with SOP, your systems may change frequently: don't worry! Changing systems is still more effective than not having a plan at all. An example of a system might be placing a trash can and a bill holder in one location near where your mail enters the house. This way, your mail can be sorted into "keep" or "toss" immediately. Examples of systems for dealing with feelings might be keeping a journal or having a friend to whom you can verbalize your overwhelming feelings. This helps reduce stress and therefore, reduce feelings of being overwhelmed.

> "When facing a difficult task act as though it is impossible to fail. If you are going after Moby Dick take along the tartar sauce."
> -Life's Little Treasure Book on Hope

Use short lists:

We recommend using a list with only one or two "to do" items on it. Bigger lists lead

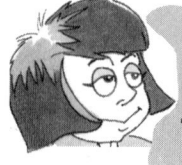

> "Challenges can be stepping stones or stumbling blocks. It's just a matter of how you view them."
>
> *-Unknown*

to bigger frustrations and feelings of being more overwhelmed.

Make a deal with yourself:

Setting an agreement and a reward for yourself can get you motivated. Saying "I'll do one load of laundry or one page of this report, then I'll give myself permission to watch a half hour of TV and zone out" sweetens the activity with the promise of a reward.

Use a master calendar:

You will not be able to remember everything. Having and using a calendar will give you a visual reminder of your goals or destinations, and therefore will cut down on your feeling overwhelmed. It's much easier to face Back to School Night when you see it coming on your calendar than when you're notified by the school with a one-day warning.

Take a mini-vacation:

Take time for yourself--even if it's a walk in the park or holing up in your bedroom with a book and your favorite music. This can reduce stress and therefore reduce feeling overwhelmed. Give yourself permission to withdraw from the chaos of life periodically in order to recover your balance. This is especially important if you've been pushing yourself to meet demands and you suddenly feel stuck.

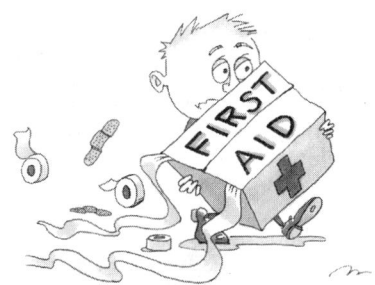

Need More First Aid?

If you are stressed about literally everything, see:
Stress Reduction in Chapter 2.

If you are feeling as though time is your enemy, see:
Time Management in

Chapter 6.

Is there is a possibility you are making things worse for yourself? If so, see: **Strategies for Death, Taxes, and Other Necessary Evils in Chapter 11.**

Do you feel as though your life is totally out of control? If so, see: **Balance in Life in Chapter 28.**

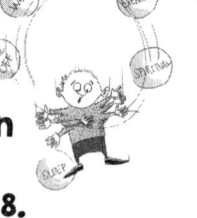

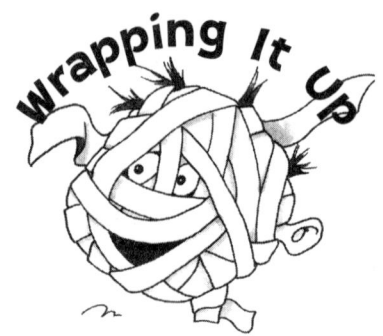

Wrapping It Up

- It is true that the world is becoming ever more complex and fast-paced.

- However, your own creativity and enthusiasm often generate your unending list of "things to do."

- Check your state of emo-

Chapter 1 • Overwhelm

tional health. Are you able to recognize patterns of depression that reduce your efficiency?

- Are you too quick to say "Yes" to anything anyone asks you to do?

- Use systems to get your life back into control.

- Recognize the feeling of being overwhelmed as a true problem, and know that you are not alone.

> "Due to our creativity and imagination, there is always one more job, one more idea, one more book to write."
> —*Joan and Denise*

Stress Reduction

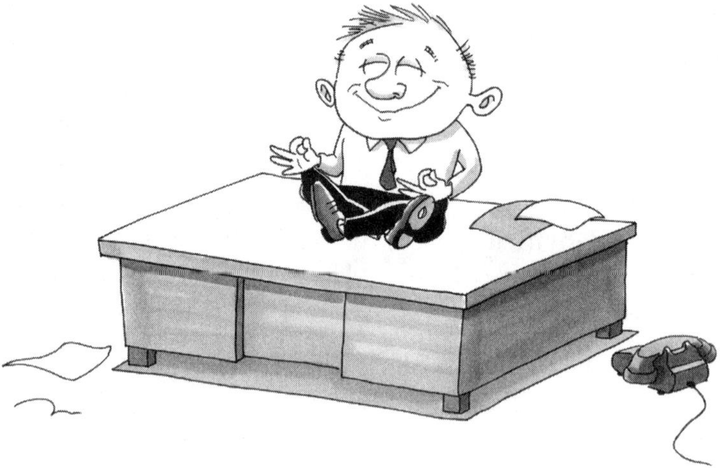

Chapter 2

What You Need To Know

Stress is a normal part of everyday life. A certain amount of stress keeps us motivated. For many AESOPs, intense surges of stress can kick us into gear and bring out the best in us. We can deliver peak performance helping out in an accident, saving the life of a child, or staying up all night to finish an important project at work. On the other hand, for the Adult with SOP, the continuous little stresses of life--balancing the checkbook, returning phone calls, making sure there is oil in the car--can do us in. Due to our unique body chemistries, when these stresses accumulate and reach a certain level there can be an actual shutdown of the brain's frontal

> "Loosen Up. Relax. Except for rare life-and-death matters nothing is as important as it first seems."
> -Life's Little Treasure Book On Wisdom

AESOP=Adults Experiencing Special Operating Problems

lobes (our decision-making area). This leaves us feeling not only overwhelmed, but also feeling as though we are falling apart and will never be able to pick up the pieces again.

The Positive Spin

Realize that for the Adult with SOP, this reaction to stress is normal. Be kinder to yourself because being hard on yourself just increases the stress. As you experiment with different techniques to deal with stress and find yourself being successful, your confidence will increase. To illustrate this, think of yourself as a driver. If you push, push, push, (careening along with pedal to the metal) you have less control when you hit a rough spot on the road. On the other hand, if you ease up on the accelerator and reduce your speed for those rough stretches of road, you'll have more control over your vehicle and the outcome of the ride.

Chapter 2 • Stress Reduction

Techniques

Breathe:

This first technique is simply remembering to breathe, slowly, calmly, and deeply under stress. We tend to tighten up, breathe very shallowly, or hold our breath when things get tough. Oxygen is a vital part of healthy body functions. A healthy body deals better with stress. Take a moment, inhale and exhale to the count of three; your whole body will respond by relaxing.

Practice switching tracks:

This technique involves breathing as well. To illustrate this, think of a train speeding down the tracks towards disaster. When the switchman sees the danger and instinctively flips the control, he redirects the train to a safer track. Under stress we are barreling down a dangerous track.

> "Breathing teaches you everything you need to know--right under your nose."
> -Gay Hendricks

We must practice switching tracks until it becomes automatic. In human terms, the switching of the tracks starts with deeper breathing. Again, oxygen is our fail-safe stress reducer. This, followed by an immediate changing of our thoughts towards a more pleasant image, brings us more quickly to reduced levels of stress.

Join a class:

Many communities provide stress-reduction or stress-management courses. They tend to be offered in evening hours or on weekends to accommodate our busy schedules. A yoga or t`ai chi class may also be helpful for stress reduction. In your exploration of these courses, look for one that focuses on the mind-body connection to make the most impact on reducing your stress.

Learn to meditate:

There are both passive and active forms of meditation. Research has proven that meditation lowers stress, pulse rate, breathing rate, and promotes relaxation and a feeling of being centered or grounded. Read one of the many books on beginning meditation, or check out the bulletin board at your local health food store for meditation coaches or classes.

Use a coach or specialist:

There are people who specialize in stress management and relaxation training. They may use tapes, environmental sounds, or hypnosis to begin to re-program you from stress-filled to stress-reduced.

Exercise:

Remember, there is no better stress reducer (with the exception of breathing) than a walk, a jog, or a swim. We live in a very busy time, and we can get so caught up in work or family obligations that we forget to take care of our bodies.

Think like a turtle:

When the world gets scary, the turtle withdraws into its shell until it is safe to emerge. Temporary periods of withdrawal are helpful for AESOPs

> "It's all right to have butterflies in your stomach. Just get them to fly in formation."
> -Dr. Rob Gilbert

AESOP=Adults Experiencing Special Operating Problems

as well. These allow us time to do an internal self-check for what we need to reduce our stress. When you're beat, take stock. Ask yourself: are you working too many hours? Are you having a disagreement with your spouse? Think carefully about your answers, and use your retreat time to begin brainstorming possible solutions from a safe place.

> *"If the stress gets too much...howl."*
> -Anne Wilson Schaef

Use an outside reality check:

Have one or two people available in your life who know you and who have good heads on their shoulders. They may be relatives, friends, counselors, or mentors. If you are currently in a pickle and don't have someone in place...get them in place for next time. Use these people's abilities to see the bigger picture in your life; have them help you decide if your perceptions are accurate when you are in the middle of a stressful situation.

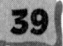

Chapter 2 • Stress Reduction

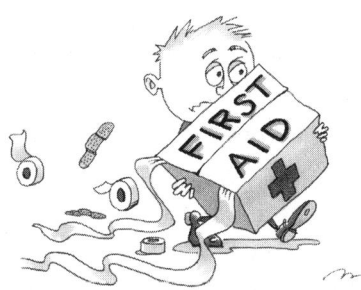

Need More First Aid?

If your stress increases because you feel like you can't handle your problems see:
Problem Solving in Chapter 3.

If you're not sure how else to reduce stress see:

Balance in Life in Chapter 28.

If you need exercise tips and ideas, see:
Exercise in Chapter 30.

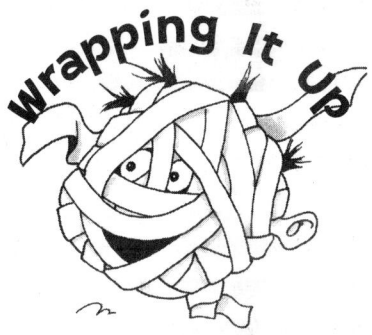

●Stress is a normal part of life. We may be able to handle the stress that major crises bring yet be completely stressed out by smaller things such as bill-paying and grocery shopping.

- Being kinder to ourselves under stress reduces it more quickly than criticizing ourselves for feeling stressed.

- Successful stress reduction and management can be achieved through a variety of techniques ranging from things we can do for ourselves to activities or people we can use as support.

> "For many AESOPs, intense surges of stress can kick us into gear and bring out the best in us. We can deliver peak performance helping out in an accident, saving the life of a child, or staying up all night to finish an important project at work."
>
> *-Joan and Denise*

AESOP=Adults Experiencing Special Operating Problems

Problem-Solving

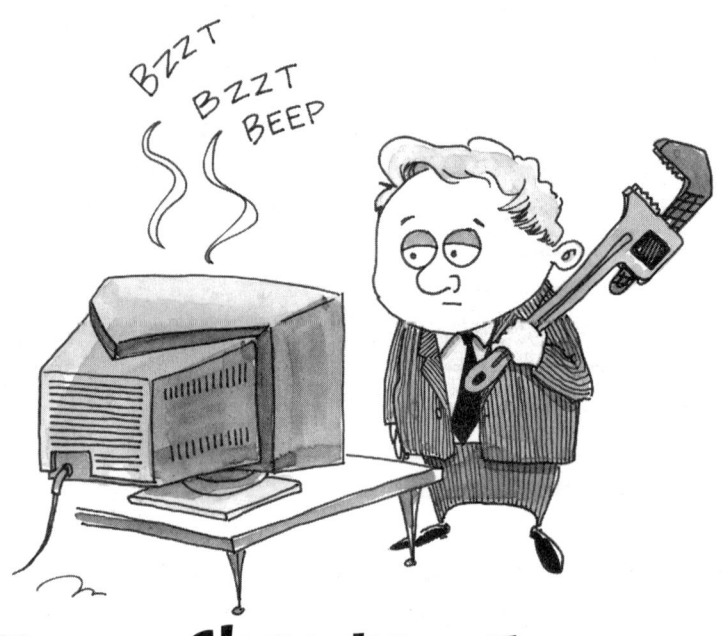

Chapter 3

What You Need To Know

Problems are a part of everyday life for the human race. For AESOPs, however, even typical problems can easily get blown out of proportion into catastrophes. In reaction to these over-inflated problems, AESOPs tend either to shut down completely and withdraw, or to jump the gun and move into action. The action response typically comes with a sense of urgency or desperation, and the feeling that something, anything at all, must be done. This frantic haste doesn't allow for a pocket of time where the Adult with SOP has time to reflect, to research facts, and to consider possible consequences for their course of action. In addition, there is typically no system put in place to provide for continuity or follow-through.

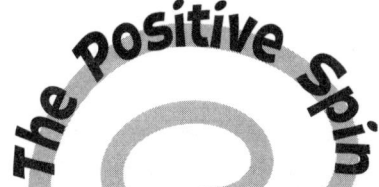

The Positive Spin

Think of life as a mosaic. As an art form, a mosaic is made up of small individual pieces

AESOP=Adults Experiencing Special Operating Problems

of ceramic or stone in varying shapes and colors. Together these individual pieces form the big picture. Our life picture is also made up of many individual elements which combine to form a whole. If part of our life picture is damaged, blemished, or broken, just like the pieces of a mosaic, it can be removed, repaired, and reinserted. Once this is accomplished, the big picture again is clear, cohesive, and unblemished.

If you are feeling that life is swirling around you, out of your control, it will help to realize that problems, like individual parts of the mosaic, can be isolated into manageable pieces.

Problem-solving is a skill that can be learned, not one of the mysteries of the universe.

Techniques

The first two techniques are actually templates. Use them to plug in specific problems and to find solutions. Don't be afraid to try both templates to find which one works best for you.

> "First ask yourself, is this my problem? If it isn't, leave it alone. If it is my problem, can I tackle it now? Do so. If your problem could be settled by an expert in some field, go quickly to him and take his advice."
>
> -Dr. Austen Riggs

Problem-Solving Template #1

Identify:

Clearly identify and define problem areas, realizing that problems are usually made up of layers. No fuzzy thinking allowed here. For example, instead of thinking, "I'm going to get fired," realize the underlying problem: "I'm late for work every day and have several pink slips." The next step is to ask yourself "Why?" which will send you researching. You might realize the deeper problem is "I can't get out of bed in the morning." You may think you are at the bottom of the problem, but press on. Why can't you get out of bed? Aha! Finally on to the "absolute" root of the problem. "I've become so desensitized to my alarms, I don't hear them ringing. Therefore, I don't get out of bed. Therefore, I'm late for work and have several pink slips. Therefore, I'm going to get fired." Finally you think you've gotten to the bottom of the problem, but did you really? There's another step to go.

Dissect:

This step requires you to delve even deeper into the root of the problem. Assess the following: Are you getting enough sleep? Is there a problem with falling asleep at night or with your overall sleep pattern? Is your body rhythm out of kilter because of school or work schedules? If none of these seem to apply, then further dissect the alarm clock situation. Are the alarms within arm's reach? Do they have snooze buttons? Is their pitch comforting rather than alarming? Is this what prevents you from getting out of bed in the morning?

> "Every problem has two handles. You can grab by the handle of fear or the handle of hope."
>
> -*Life's Little Treasure Book On Hope*

Create:

The final step is to create a solution. Give yourself permission to be creative and innovative in this phase. Realize that the first solution may not work, and that you may need to stair-step one solution on top of another. Here's a case study which illustrates the creativity of a good solution. A single woman client was on the verge of getting fired because she truly was no longer able to hear any of her three alarm clocks, (including the one she had positioned across the room in a metal pail for added racket). Her next move was to arrange for two separate wake-up services to call her with a live voice at the other end of the phone. However, within a month she found that she could answer the call, sound coherent and fall back asleep. Her final solution, after much researching, was to buy a state-of-the-art, vibrating alarm clock (typically used for the hearing impaired), which shook her awake each morning.

Problem-Solving Template #2

Define the problem:

You must grasp and clearly understand your problem. If you're having trouble seeing the problem clearly, try putting it on paper or talking it through with a friend. For example, you are enrolled in college classes and are afraid that you won't make it through the semester. You're falling behind in several of your subjects and you've had several absences. The specific problem to solve would be "What are my options with respect to my classes?"

Brainstorm:

This step requires you to think creatively, to develop possible solutions, considering even the ones that seem improbable. This is not a place to limit yourself; at times,

> "I'm grateful for all my problems. As each of them was overcome I became stronger and more able to meet those yet to come. I grew on my difficulties."
>
> —J.C. Penney

the solution that seems improbable might fit you best. For example, in brainstorming you may write down options such as getting a tutor, dropping a class, quitting school, getting a minimum wage job, cutting classes to avoid the problem, or marrying the first eligible person that comes along to get yourself out of the rat race. Once you've allowed your mind to develop all of the possibilities, take an honest look at your options and cross off the ones that are truly improbable.

Identify pros and cons:

Take each of the remaining probable solutions and write a list of pros and cons.

Select one:

Choose the solution that

appears most likely to succeed based on your lists of pros and cons.

Do it:

This step may involve simply putting your solution into action. If your solution is complex, involving several steps, list Step 1, Step 2, and so on. Give yourself a reasonable time frame that you'll dedicate to this solution before moving on to the next step.

Evaluate:

Without taking it personally, look at whether your plan or solution is working. If it's working, great, leave it alone and continue. If it's not working, go back to "Select One" and choose another likely option.

Miscellaneous Stuff about Problem-Solving

Research:

Looking further into the problem typically takes two directions in the AESOP world. In one direction, the AESOP avoids research entirely. In the opposite direction, the AESOP develops tunnel vision and

> "Problems are like a box of crackerjacks. If you look closely enough you will always find the prize."
>
> *-Life's Little Treasure Book On Hope*

researches ad nauseum without ever solving the problem. To find the middle ground, use the rule of three: Get three different opinions, get three different sources (don't forget the Internet), get three different quotes, and then get going! Remember to give yourself a time limit to complete this step.

Evaluate:

Step back; take a clear look at what's working for you and what's not. Adults with SOP tend to take problems or "failures" in very personal terms. Distance yourself and approach this as a problem-solving exercise, not as a personal judgment of your self-worth.

24-Hour Rule:

Do you find yourself impulsively jumping to the first possible solution? Stop. Make a firm rule for yourself that you'll allow 24 hours before stepping forward with a decision. When dealing with other people, cultivate phrases like "Let me think about that; I'll get back to you tomorrow." Or "I'd like to do a little research on this; let me get back to you tomorrow."

Freeze Frame:

If you catch yourself going off on a wild goose chase or about to make an impulsive decision...FREEZE! Imagine a film stopped at one frame. This allows you to examine the action and its consequences in detail. Ask yourself if this picture is going to have a good ending. At this point you may choose to rewind the film and try again.

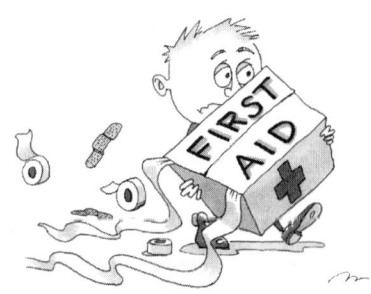

Need More First Aid?

If you are having trouble even beginning to research

possible solutions to your problems, see:
Procrastination in Chapter 6.

Do you start something only to fizzle out rather quickly? Take a look at:
Consistency in Chapter 8.

Do you constantly beat yourself up for your failures? You might need help in dealing with shame and guilt. If so check out:
Shame and Guilt in Chapter 18.

Is the world totally overwhelming? Do you feel as though you are in deep water and going down for the third time? Where do you derive your support? Look up:
Chapter 34 on Spirituality.

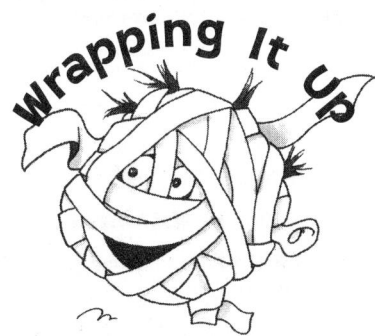

●Problems are to be expected

in the normal course of our lives.

- For AESOPs, problems too often cause a sense of panic.

- Panic often leads to a feeling of urgency, which results in hasty decisions.

- It is important to slow down the process.

- Each problem can be isolated, the root cause identified, and corrections made.

- Once this is accomplished, the corrected problem becomes a repaired piece of our life, which can be then plugged back into the big picture.

> "Realize that problems, like individual parts of the mosaic, can be isolated into manageable pieces. Problem-solving is a skill that can be learned, not one of the mysteries of the universe."
>
> *-Joan and Denise*

AESOP=Adults Experiencing Special Operating Problems

Organization

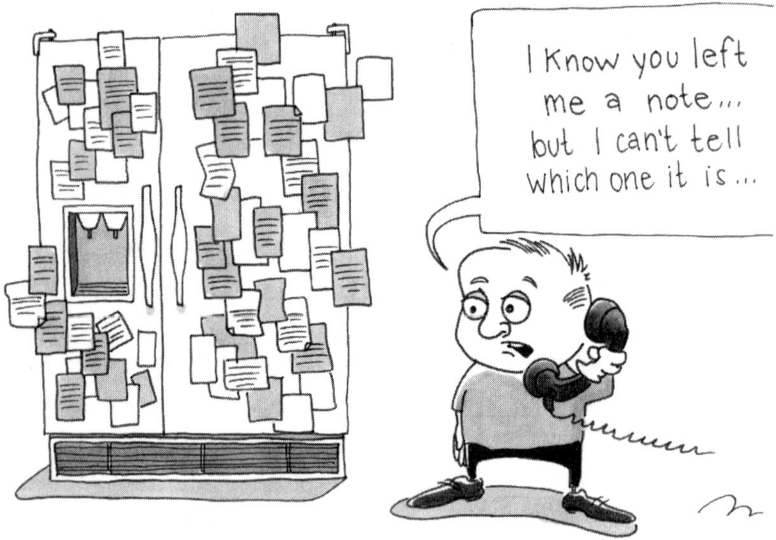

Chapter 4

What You Need To Know

Although AESOPs may have a constant commitment to getting organized, actually doing it and maintaining it can be an AESOP's nightmare. For every system put in place to keep one thing organized--outgoing bills, for example--another three are needed to find missing stamps, car keys, and tools. We can put system after system of organization into place, but we fall to pieces when these systems have to be maintained with consistency (another AESOP's nightmare!).

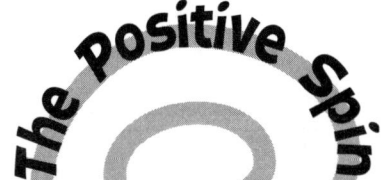

The Positive Spin

As creative and innovative adults, we often invent or design systems that work very well; the trouble is, we only maintain them for a short period of time. Once we find that our marvelous systems have fallen apart, we discard them and never give them a second chance. We need to realize that the flaw is probably not with

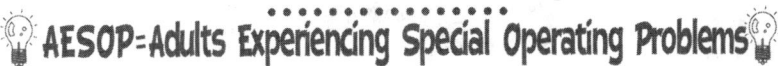

AESOP=Adults Experiencing Special Operating Problems

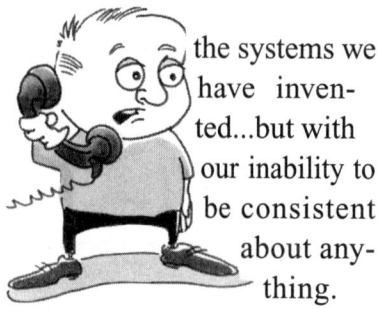
the systems we have invented...but with our inability to be consistent about anything.

Remember, our wonderful qualities of spontaneity and innovation predispose us to be intermittent rather than consistent. The ability to be consistent is typically not in an AESOP's nature. The old saying, "If it ain't broke, don't fix it" can take on a new meaning here. Think back: was there once a really effective way to remember your keys, glasses, and important papers? It's OK to go back to what worked before and re-implement that organizational system. In fact, it's possible to go back to an old system many times, dust it off, polish it a bit, and use it again.

Techniques
Use People to Help

Use a friend:

Many times our friends are AESOPs too, and are just as unorganized as we are. Because there is a common link (the mutually shared AESOP condi-

Chapter 4 • Organization

tion), these friends provide you a safe place to admit your need for help without embarrassment. Even so, choose the friends for this technique carefully. Make sure they are empathetic and kind. Once this is done, the next step is to verbalize your need to get organized and ask for their help. The next step is to brainstorm some possible strategies (and believe us, it works better with more than one brain!). Finally, ask your friend to play a supportive role as you work on your organization. Ask them to praise you when you are successful and support you when you are floundering as you attempt to refine the perfect strategy.

Use an organized friend:

If you are lucky enough to have either an AESOP friend who falls at the compulsive end of the continuum or an organized non-AESOP friend, you are in luck. Getting such a friend to spend an hour or two helping you organize can motivate you and make the process less lonely. Whether you work with a friend or by yourself, here's a tip: be sure to focus on a specific area you want to organize. If your plans are too global, you'll get overwhelmed and feel discouraged, with or without a friend.

Use a professional organizer:

If you are truly organizationally challenged, consider hiring someone whose specialty is getting others organized. Professional organizers know how to approach a mess with a skilled eye on how to turn that disaster into a workable system.

Hire other help:

If you are organizationally challenged to the max, turn the entire mess over to someone else. Hire part-time help to pay

> "If your aim is control, it must be self-control first. If your aim is management, it must be self-management first."
>
> *-Anonymous*

your bills, keep your files organized, and keep you on track. It is well worth the small amount of money you will spend. AESOPs who are aware of their shortcomings may marry someone who is super-organized and solve their problems that way. Often this occurs with no prior plan, but if you are making a list of things you want in a mate, organization might be high on the list!

Consider Organizational Tricks
Think containment:

Don't let those scraps of paper, receipts, or notes from your child's teacher disappear into your car trunk or get lost on the garage workbench. Buy a big basket, a large trash can, or anything else that can stay in one spot in your house. Choose something that will hold a bunch of "stuff." Train yourself to put everything in this one spot. You won't lose anything vital this way. At a pre-set interval once or twice a month, empty your basket or trash can on the floor or table. Next, choose categories for sorting. One might be "school stuff," others might be "bills to pay," "income tax," "stuff to throw away," and don't forget "miscellaneous" for those items that defy categorization. Write each category on a large piece of paper with a black marking pen and lay the paper on the floor. Gather up the stack of stuff in your arm and walk down the row of categories, sorting your bits of paper into piles as you go. After everything is sorted, take care of immediate issues such as writing checks to pay bills, signing your child's field trip permission slip, etc. Then, move the remaining piles into another holding area. The next step for a category like "income taxes" may be an even larger basket in a closet where all your tax material is kept. "School stuff" might go in an accordion file that you may (or may not) sort through later, and so on. The goal is to completely empty your basket. The process is then started again.

> "The art of progress is to preserve order amid change, and to preserve change amid order."
> -A.N. Whitehead

It may not look pretty, but it's really quite efficient, and you won't lose anything crucial.

Allow time for organizing:

We make appointments to get our hair cut or to take our dog to the vet. If we don't plan ahead, these things either don't get done or we lose valuable time sitting in the waiting room fuming. In this same way, we need to plan time in our days so that we can get organized. Organization doesn't just happen for AESOPs. Shoot for an hour a day to organize, make lists, return phone calls, and plan your schedule.

Narrow your focus:

Looking at the total mess is overwhelming, whether it is an entire room in chaos or a desk that is buried under stacks of papers. Focus on just one thing and keep at it until that one thing is completed. This might mean that your first job is to pick up all the toys and articles of clothing strewn around the living room. Do that first, and do it completely! Stop. Praise yourself. Then jump back in and tackle the second job.

Everything must have its place:

Part of what makes organizing so difficult is the question "Well, where am I going to put it?" It is essential that you identify, create, or build a place for the things you're organizing. More than half the battle is knowing where to put things back after you use them.

Some examples are:

- keys in a basket by the back door
- wallet or purse on the dresser in the bedroom
- glasses on the desk
- cell phone in your purse (female)
- cell phone with your wallet (male)
- notes from children's teachers in basket on the desk
- check to be deposited on refrigerator door and secured by a huge magnetic clip
- items to go to work tomorrow put under your purse or under your shoes
- recipes in one drawer, all

Chapter 4 • Organization

in one place to be re-filed (one day)

- dog leash hooked by back door

Use labeled accordion files:

Whether you label by topic (car, mortgage, utilities) or by name (clients Smith, Jones, Washington), having specific titles on your files helps you stay organized.

Create order within your system:

Even though repetition is hard for many AESOPs, it also helps keep a structure. Let's use tackling the mail as an example. In establishing a system to organize your mail, you need a stacking tray for bills, a trash can or recycling bin for unwanted mailers and catalogs, a place for personal notes which need answering, and an area for "I should read this when I have time." A chair or counter top close by your usual entrance point to the house is recommended, especially if you get a lot of mail. Organize your trays and bins from left to right or vice-versa, and do not vary

> "It wasn't raining when Noah built the ark."
> -Howard Ruff

their function. Soon your brain will accept the order and things will become much smoother and more automatic. Again, do not change your system, or you'll have to start all over again.

Need More First Aid?

If the need to organize your time prevents you from organizing anything else, see:
Time Management in Chapter 5

If putting things off is a problem, see:
Procrastination in Chapter 6.

If clutter is a big part of your organizing difficulties, check out:
Clutter in Chapter 7

Wrapping It Up

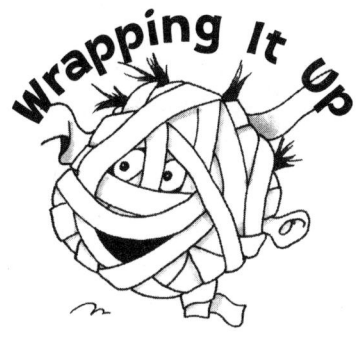

- Getting organized requires a consistent and constant effort.

- You don't just "get organized," you forever work at remaining organized.

- Remember, old systems you have discarded may be excellent. Take them out, dust them off, and try them again.

- Don't be afraid to turn to other people to help you organize.

- Rest easy. There are a multitude of techniques that you can plug in to solve your organizational problems.

- Most important of all, trust yourself. You do have the capability to contain the chaos in your life!

> "Out of clutter, find simplicity."
> *-Albert Einstein*

Time Management

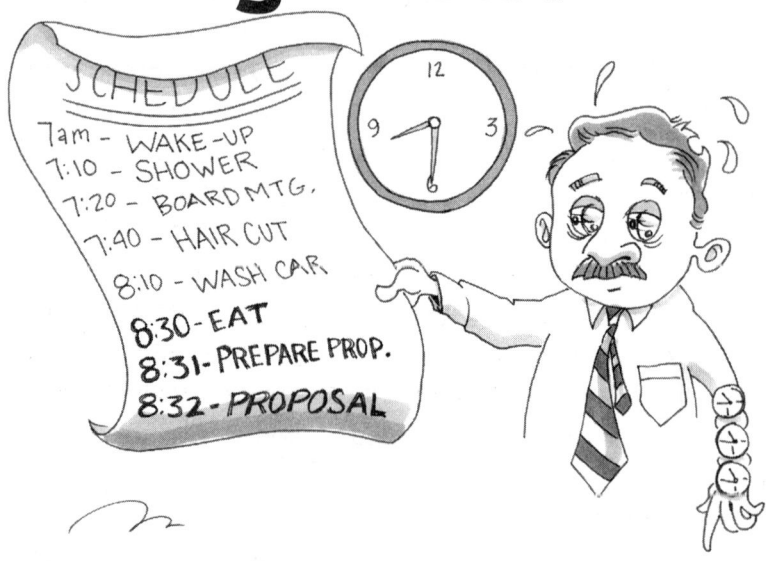

Chapter 5

What You Need To Know

Adults with SOP typically have marvelous ideas percolating in our very busy brains as well as lists of things we'd love to get done. The problem is there just never seems to be enough time. Even when time is available, figuring out what to do first, second, and third feels overwhelming. Then there are those dull, routine tasks such as bill-paying, washing the dishes, or doing our taxes that weigh on us like albatrosses around our necks.

For the AESOP, time is like a rubber band. The rubber band--our sense of time--may stretch out to the limit; we feel as though we have all the time in the world to complete a particular job or finally check off all the items on our list. The trouble is, we often feel there is so much time that we add even more to our list. Alternately, we may be lulled into a sense of complacency and put off doing anything at all for another day. The end result is that things don't get done.

On the other hand, our rubber

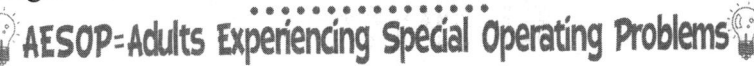

AESOP=Adults Experiencing Special Operating Problems

> "Time is what we want most, but, what, alas, we use worst."
> —*William Penn*

band may feel very constrictive, as though it is wound up tight. At those times, we experience tremendous pressure and a sick feeling in the pit of our stomachs--we've taken on too much--again. We know there is no time to get everything done. At those times, the AESOP typically shuts down; we are feeling so overwhelmed that we are immobilized. Again, the end result is that nothing gets done.

To add to the complexities of managing time, the nature of our AESOP body chemistry may in fact, be responsible for giving us an altered concept of time. While the rest of the world is operating on "real time," our world is operating on "AESOP time." This can cause problems because people in the "real world" may see us as "flaky" or unresponsive to the needs of others.

The Positive Spin

We need to embrace our uniqueness and creativity. The thousands of thoughts that race through our minds, the endless list of projects we devise, are gifts. Wouldn't life be boring if we had absolutely nothing we wanted to do? We just need to be conscious of our time management. Here is a twofold solution. First, we must get a grip on what happens to us when we have either too much or too little time. Second, we must develop techniques for managing our own particular type of "AESOP time." Remember, the tools and techniques are very specific; what works well for one AESOP might not work for another. Above all, the goal is to manage our time. In accomplishing this goal, we shouldn't feel guilty about the lengths to which we need to go. Every time we manage time successfully, no matter how we do it, we win!

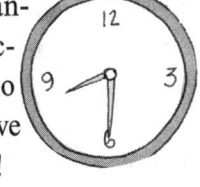

AESOP=Adults Experiencing Special Operating Problems

Techniques
Tools for Your Toolbox

Think of this first set of techniques as tools for a toolbox that you develop and carry with you, much as a plumber or carpenter does. These tools are as important to the AESOP as a pipe wrench is to a plumber or a saw is to a carpenter.

Master Calendar:

This is for you and your entire family. It should be kept in plain sight at all times such as on the refrigerator.

- Keep all your personal appointments listed, such as doctor's appointments and Back to School Night, preferably using colored markers, so things don't get booked on top of each other.

- Update your calendar weekly.

- You must run the calendar, not the other way around. Remember to schedule free time; you must decide when to take a weekend off. If you don't, your life will get so full you'll never take time for yourself.

- List all birthdays, anniversaries, religious ceremonies

Chapter 5 • Time Management

for your family and friends. That way you will have a chance of keeping yourself out of trouble.

● At the end of the year, move all the important events to your new calendar. Be sure to schedule this task. It can even become part of your New Year's traditions; how about doing it while you watch the Rose Parade? Remember, if you don't identify a specific time to break out your new calendar, it will never happen.

Day-Planner:

This can be manual, electronic, or computerized. Different systems work for different people. Keep trying until you find the best fit for yourself. Bits and pieces of information as well as receipts and little scraps of paper often get put in a day-planner. Consider purchasing a day-planner that zips shut or has lots of pockets.

● Log incoming and outgoing calls.

● Log daily appointments.

● Make a tickler file for something you'd like to accomplish the next day.

• Keep running lists of goals you'd like to accomplish.

Timer:

This can range from a watch to an electronic kitchen timer. We've already identified our "different" conceptualization of time; this helps us monitor it. Set the timer for a specific amount of time to accomplish a task. When the timer goes off, either move on to another task or re-negotiate to give the task a few more minutes. Either way, this reminds us not to let time run away.

Electronic Warning System:

From a five-alarm watch to a beep from our personal electronic notebook, an electronic warning system alerts us that something is imminent. This can be used to time medica-

> "Whatever the right hand findeth to do, the left hand carries a watch on its wrist to show how long it takes to do it."
>
> -Ralph W. Sockmon

Chapter 5 • Time Management

tion, or to trigger us to get on the road, pick up our child, or show up at an important business appointment. Note: sometimes we need a "pre-warning beep," a "warning beep," and then the "real beep" to get us moving.

Post-its©:

There are a multitude of uses for these little gems:

- Write specific appointment times on a post-it© and put it on your steering wheel or computer screen to jog your memory and keep you on time and on task.

- Write one post-it© note for each of the things you need to do. You can arrange these in order of priority. There's a great satisfaction in throwing them away when you are finished with each task.

- Post-its© can be used to label stacks of papers or stacks of files that you've reviewed with instructions such as "File under X in drawer," or "Complete by X date." This saves you the time of going back through something you've already done.

- Use a post-it© on your bills to warn you to pay by a certain date. (A due date for a bill can also be reflected on your master calendar).

Boxes, shopping bags, large receptacles:

If you are working on a project that is multi-faceted, keep everything that is related in one place. Six shopping bags stored in a corner may not be pretty, but the information needed for the project is contained and accessible. This not only saves time, but ensures that you won't lose anything vital.

Secretary:

In addition to preparing your toolbox, consider finding an assistant. The trick is to enlist the help of someone who is better at managing a calendar than you are. This could be your significant other or someone you specifically hire for the job. This someone might do routine tasks, such as taking clothes to the cleaners or dropping things at the post office; they might also pay the bills or organize your paperwork for the day. The ultimate secretary is a person (or a service) who takes care of birthdays and important events, and lets everyone know you are the caring and loving person that you truly are (under all that paperwork).

Ideas for Managing Time

Be realistic:

Realize that as an Adult with SOP, you will NEVER be able to complete everything. New ideas will keep popping up, and your list will be endless. Therefore, concentrate on doing one or two things on your list each day, not on finishing the list.

Make a general list:

Write down where your time goes each week. Don't forget to include routine, but necessary, things like showering, driving to work, working out, and making meals. From that master list decide if it's even possible for you to do the things you have planned. Realize that it may be necessary to hire someone to take some of the load off your shoulders.

Use a system:

Frequently, AESOPs have trouble with time management and priorities because we take care of things as they come up, rather than having a system to decide what should be taken care of first, second, or third. We may sit down to study chemistry only to be distracted by a loose pile of papers threatening to fall off the desk, then be drawn toward the bookshelves to re-organize them, then be driven to go next door to borrow our neighbor's hedge trimmer. The following A-B-C priority system is designed to help us look at our "to do" list, assign a priority status to each item or activity, and complete the important items on our list.

The A-B-C System:

Make an on-going list of chores, tasks, projects.

If a project is lengthy or involved, such as painting the house, break it into smaller discrete pieces. For example, your list would read: sand trim, blast eaves, repair termite damage, buy paint, paint stucco, paint trim, and finally, clean up job and put all tools away.

Look at your list and assign each item that you *must* do (or

> "Next week there can't be any crisis. My schedule is already full."
> -Henry Kissinger

the world will fall apart) with the letter A.

Next we move right to the "C's" on our list because they are easy to identify. Scan your list and target the items that would be wonderful to have done, but truly aren't earth-shaking. Mark these with the letter "C." An example of a "C" item would be to put photos in a photo album, or to separate the box of screws and nails in the garage into different containers.

Move all the other items into the "B" category. "B's" are essentially items that ultimately will move up to the "A" category as you knock off "A's" and re-prioritize.

Each time you add an item to the list, give it an "A," "B," or "C."

The UNBREAKABLE rule that will make this system work: you must complete one "A" each and every day. Just think, by the end of the month you'll have 30 or 31 "A's" completed! By the end of the year, with 365 "A's" crossed off your list, you'll feel like you are the most organized person in the world.

Check your master calendar:

At the beginning of each month, check for all upcoming events. Make one trip to the mall and purchase cards and gifts needed for the entire month. Come home and promptly wrap and mail them. It's OK to be a little ahead for once! Your friends and family will be impressed beyond belief with your thoughtfulness.

Clear ample time:

This one requires pulling out your day-planner, calendar or computer calendar again (attempting to retain your schedule in your head sets you up to forget what you need to remember). Decide what you want to accomplish. Identify the specific action needed and describe it as simply and directly as possible: wash car, read two chapters, write memo to staff. Allot adequate time for each goal, then add some additional time. The added time allows for traffic, malfunctioning equipment, and delays. If you fall off schedule even when clearing ample time,

> "Don't say you don't have enough time. You have exactly the same number of hours per day that were given to Helen Keller, Louis Pasteur, Michelangelo, Mother Teresa, Thomas Jefferson, and Albert Einstein."
>
> -*Life's Little Treasure Book On Success*

give yourself five minutes to be upset with yourself, then analyze what broke down. Was my system too complicated? Did I understand how long certain tasks would take? Did I get distracted and lose track of time? Now start again!

Clump necessary items:

Identify the project. List all the items needed. Be complete and comprehensive in your list; a brainstorming technique is often helpful here. If you need to buy an item at the hardware or stationery store, do it BEFORE you start the project. If you miss this step and need to stop in the middle of your project to buy a crucial item, you are in trouble. Once you are out of the house it is too easy to think of other things you really need to do "while you're out," such as stopping at the cleaners and the grocery store. Inevitably, by the time you get home it will be too late to get back into your project. The rule is: clump everything you will need for the project before you begin. Using your list, concentrate on the single purpose of clumping everything in one place--hurry, hurry, hurry! If you stop to think about anything else but getting everything into one place, you'll get sidetracked. We know from experience.

Use a Distraction List:

We waste a lot of time being distracted by the things we'd like to do or need to do that we're currently not doing; we worry about outside things because we're afraid we'll forget them. Place a piece of paper clearly labeled "Distraction List" at the side of your project. Write any distracting thoughts there for later reference. This allows you to concentrate on the task at hand. When the task at hand is done, you can go back to your distraction list and decide if any of those items need action.

Always have Plan B:

The best laid plans, especially those made by AESOPs, often fall short. Always have a backup plan that leaves you still feeling as if you've accomplished something with your time. If installing a sprinkler line in your backyard is "Plan A," "Plan B" might be to complete it on just the south side of the house.

Be prepared to slide right into "Plan B" with no regrets:

Don't hang on to a "Plan A" that is not working. Although the problem may come from underestimating the time needed or as a result of forgetting to use a technique, it may also be due to things completely beyond your control such as rain, a broken water line, or your mother dropping

AESOP=Adults Experiencing Special Operating Problems

in unexpectedly. Be willing to move on to "Plan B." It's as though you are moving through a maze and you come to a dead end. You need to move quickly into an alternate route without missing a beat. It's OK to move to "Plan B." Leaving "Plan A" is not a failure.

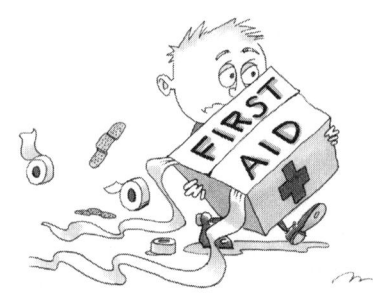

Need More First Aid?

If you have too many things on your plate and your life is overflowing, check out: **Overwhelm in Chapter 1.**

If your surroundings are in chaos, the place to

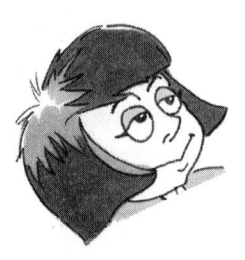

Chapter 5 • Time Management

start might be:
Chapter 7 on Clutter

Do things in your world such as noise, interruptions, or bright colors crowd your brain and make organizing your time impossible? If so, read:
Chapter 10 on Distractibility.

Do you have good intentions, but typically shoot yourself in the foot? You might find some answers in:
Chapter 13 on Self-Sabotage.

If your spouse or significant other accuses you of not caring because you have forgotten their birthday again, read:
Chapter 21, Help For Yourself in a Relationship.

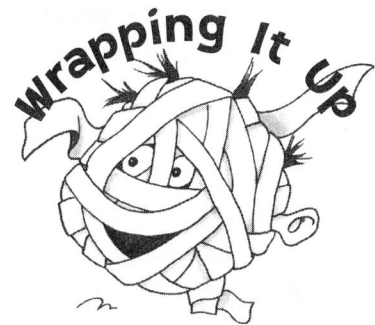

●AESOPs are often wonderfully creative and have

endless lists of projects and things they want to do.

● Unfortunately, time management often becomes a problem. AESOPs typically have a sense of either too much or too little time in which to complete things. Either of these realizations creates problems for the AESOP, and too often, nothing gets done.

● With a list of tools for time management as well as suggestions for specific techniques, the road becomes clear.

● Creativity and non-linear thinking as we problem-solve this area lead to success.

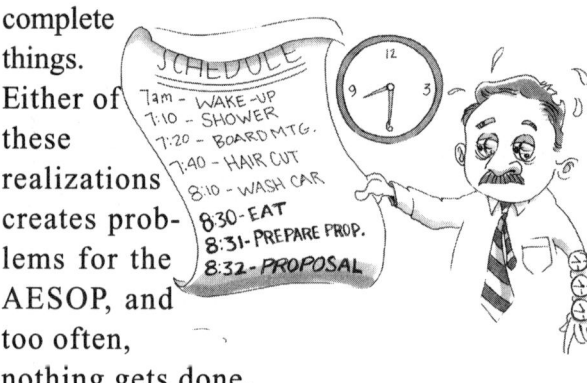

Chapter 5 • Time Management

> "Above all, the goal is to manage our time. In accomplishing this goal, we shouldn't feel guilty about the lengths to which we need to go. Every time we manage time successfully, no matter how we do it, we win!"
>
> *-Joan and Denise*

AESOP=Adults Experiencing Special Operating Problems

Procrastination

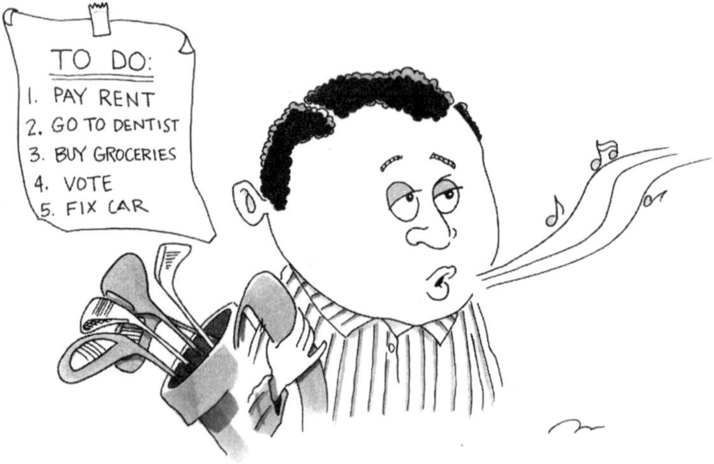

Chapter 6

What You Need To Know

Procrastination is the middle name of many AESOPs. "I'll start the paperwork tomorrow." "Just let me finish my coffee, and then I'll dust the mini blinds." We have good intentions, but poor follow-through. Did you ever wonder why? Usually the job isn't too hard. That isn't the reason at all.

Often procrastination occurs because the Adults with SOP can't muster up enough energy to jump over the imagined barrier and actually begin the project.

Complicating matters are the nearly inevitable feelings of guilt. Once procrastination is established as a pattern, guilt for all the things forever left undone tugs and pulls at the edges of our minds. This guilt combines

> "Opportunity is missed by most people because it is dressed in overalls and looks like work." *-Thomas Edison*

AESOP=Adults Experiencing Special Operating Problems

with feelings of "What is wrong with me?" to slow us down even more.

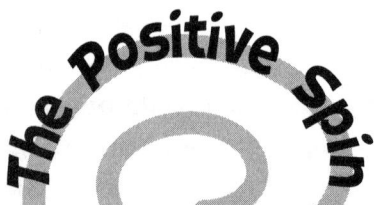
The Positive Spin

Being a procrastinator doesn't make you a bad person. Too often we apply a moral judgment to the procrastination which adds to our paralysis. Step back, and see procrastination as a behavior that can be identified and tamed. For AESOPs with difficulty facing tasks, procrastination can be a coping mechanism.

In fact, waiting until the last minute (or procrastinating) can increase the adrenaline flow and actually result in an incredible end product.

Techniques
Be real!

If you continue to procrastinate, you will feel crummy about yourself no matter how you attempt to excuse your actions. Recognize that beginning and sticking with a project will make you feel better. The alternative, avoiding any action, will leave you with that nagging feeling of pressure and worry always in the back of your mind.

Handle routine paperwork by setting a deadline for yourself:

Take control by setting a deadline for yourself, rather than hanging back and having this deadline imposed on you by someone else. Commit to your boss or spouse that something will be done by a specific date. If you have a proposal in the works but can't get it off the ground, call a meeting BEFORE the proposal is complete. Promise the five people you have asked to attend the meeting that the proposal will be ready for their review. The concept of setting your own deadline allows you to manage even routine paperwork or tasks and puts control back in your hands. Drawing other people into that deadline serves as a motivating commitment to meet the mark.

Calendar each project:

Use your monthly calendar to schedule each part of a project and its completion date. This means being able to break your projects into parts.

Separate Parts:

Look at the entire project, and conceptualize how you can separate it into manageable parts. For example, your taxes are due, and you have a year's worth of bills and receipts in front of you. First, sort them into piles labeled: House, Business Expenses, Contributions, Child Care, etc. Lay each category on the floor in a clear space. Grab the pile of jumbled paperwork in your arm and walk down the row of categories, dropping each piece of paperwork onto its appropriate spot. Once the paperwork is sorted, tackle one pile at a time, tallying, pitching, filing. Before you realize it, the job is done.

Watch out for overloading your schedule:

Filling your day too full gives you a good excuse never to begin that project. Be reasonable with your to-do list. Adults with SOP tend to have lists that go on and on and on. Realize a day. If this sounds too "easy," consider this--keep to this concept of one project a day, and

> "God put me on this planet to accomplish a certain number of things. Right now I'm so far behind, I will never die."
>
> *-Anonymous*

that you will always have something you want or need to do. And don't wait to begin an important new project until you have completed your current list. It will never happen!

Do one thing at a time:

Identify JUST ONE PROJECT that you will complete in a day. you will have 365 projects done in a year. Wow! Pretty exciting for all of us procrastinators.

Handle tedious projects and reward yourself:

Break the project into parts. Complete one part, and then reward yourself. (If I type two pages, I'll have a cup of coffee.)

Give yourself a big reward after the full project is done. This may even include a day off to do nothing at all. The trick is to line up your next project so that procrastination doesn't creep in again.

Identify stalling strategies:

We sometimes find ourselves dreading a project, saying to ourselves, "The job is too big!". Often the task can seem huge, even though you know you have the capability to do it, and do it well. Often this is "FEAR": False Evidence Appearing Real. FEAR may be the actual culprit. Ask yourself, "What am I saying to myself to stall the project?". Stalling can occur not only at

> "When there is a hill to climb, don't think that waiting will make it smaller."
> -Life's Little Treasure Book on Wisdom

the beginning of a project, but also in the middle or toward the end. Once you can identify what you're saying to yourself, such as, "This is taking forever," "I don't know what to do next," or "I think I'm in over my head," you've made a good start. Now you can look for a small thread to begin to unravel the larger ball of yarn.

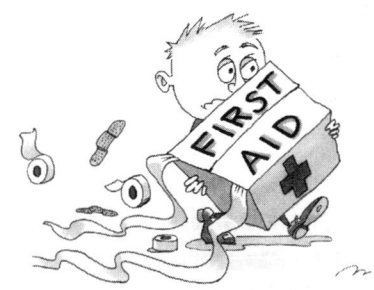

Need More First Aid?

If the world seems just too much to contemplate, check out:
Overwhelm in Chapter 1.

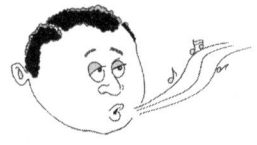

If you feel totally stressed

AESOP=Adults Experiencing Special Operating Problems

out, check out:
Stress Reduction in Chapter 2.

If you have trouble with scheduling time, read about:
Time Management in Chapter 5.

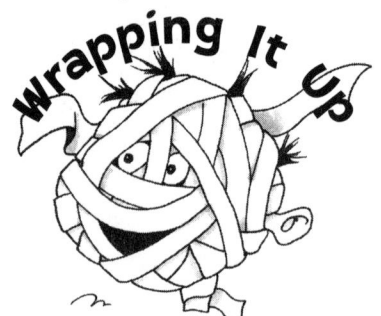

Wrapping It Up

- Procrastination brings with it feelings of shame and guilt, which lead to even more procrastination.

- Remind yourself that procrastination is not a moral issue or a character flaw.

- Some simple coping techniques can do a lot to reduce procrastination and put you back in control.

Chapter 6 • Procrastination

> "Don't give up. Keep going. There is always a chance that you will stumble onto something terrific. I have never heard of anyone stumbling over anything while he was sitting down."
>
> *-Ann Landers*

Clutter

Chapter 7

What You Need To Know

Clutter is accumulating all over the house and office! Stacks and stacks and piles and piles seem to have a life of their own (and a definite ability to generate more and more paper). Clutter can grow into an overwhelming obstacle in your life. This phenomenon is a horror for many SOP Adults.

> "Stacks and stacks and piles and piles seem to have a life of their own."
> *-Joan and Denise*

The Positive Spin

Being a clutterer is a genetic trait. It will stick with you like Velcro, so don't plan to erase the tendency from your personality profile. After all, antique shops, museums, and archives all over the world exist because of people like you! Instead, for your own peace of mind, work out a system of containment.

AESOP=Adults Experiencing Special Operating Problems

Techniques

Break the surface tension:

When clutter reaches a certain level, the amount of shame and guilt that sets in is often immobilizing. To break the surface tension and allow some clearing to occur, ask a trusted friend who is understanding and non-judgmental to help you with the first step of organizing or disposing of your treasures.

Learn to see the clutter:

We can become "house blind" or "office blind" and truly not see the clutter as others see it. Enlisting another person to work with you helps you to see your space through another's eyes. Again, the person must be non-judgmental. Just their presence can be enough to allow you clarity.

Plan your attack:

Different AESOPs need individual approaches to attacking a clutter problem. Some can only handle 10 minutes at a time as they sort through items and papers they cherish.

For them, a longer time creates too much emotional strain. For others, once they begin, they move into a type of overdrive (until they reach exhaustion). Their systems will work better if they keep on until they have completed their goal.

> "Be an original. If that means being a little eccentric, so be it."
> -*Life's Little Treasure Book On Wisdom*

Keep the 10 Minute rule:

If ten minutes is your limit, use a timer to mark the beginning and the end of each segment. Promise yourself that you will work diligently during the 10 minutes and then take 5 minutes (also using a timer) for a sip of coffee or a quick walk outside.

Use the idea of clumping:

If you are attacking a large amount of clutter, make sure that you have everything necessary to complete the job before you start. For example, you may need to visit the stationery store and buy felt markers, boxes with lids, folders, packing tape, post it© notes, accordion files, a stapler, and paper clips. Let's be real. As an AESOP Adult, if you begin this task and find that you need to make a "quick" run to the stationery store, you will actually stop at the grocery store, the cleaners, and the bookstore before you return home. Finally, you will convince yourself that it is too late to begin attacking clutter that day anyway.

Practice sorting:

You have a mound of paperwork. To attack it, first take an 8½"x11" sheet of paper. With a felt pen, write several general categories, one to a page that will cover the material in your mound. Be sure to include "miscellaneous" or its better-named twin "I don't know where this belongs." Don't forget a pile for recycling. Dis-tribute these large pieces of paper on the living room floor. Grab an armful from your mound. Walk down the row of categories, dropping each piece of paper onto its appropriate pile.

Once the mound is distributed, it's now decision time. Some of the piles might need to be stored in a carefully marked box and put in the closet or the garage. Some of the stacks might need to be further sorted into separate categories. For example, if one stack is labeled "Bills" it might be sorted into the following: Bills to Pay, Bills to File, Bills for Tax Records. The very act of sorting begins to organize our clutter.

Contain newspapers and magazines:

The printed page holds such delicious ideas for that intriguing recipe you want to try or a new bathroom treatment that would be wonderful. With an AESOP's often poor memory, you just know you will never remember your current inspiration in the future. So what do you do? You save the entire paper or magazine, usually in a pile of other papers or magazines that you know have something important in them, somewhere. Try this: buy a box that will hold scissors, tape, stapler, pens, and articles that you'll cut out. Keep this wherever you normally read your paper or maga-

> "When in doubt, throw it out."
> -Anonymous

zines. Pro-mise yourself that if you see a neat idea you will cut it out immediately and then THROW OUT the rest of the the newspaper or magazine. The precious article goes in the bottom of the box, saved, but taking up much less space. For the avid saver, consider reducing the number of magazine or newspaper subscriptions that arrive at your door.

Contain photos and keepsakes:

In our lives, there will always be items such as photos, programs from our kids' school events, and special cards or notes that we want to keep. This is OK, but once again the idea is containment. Arrange a spot in a closet where boxes can be kept dry and safe from insects. Purchase boxes with lids. Pile keepsakes and photos in a box until it is full. Seal and date the box. Some day, when you are retired and have all the time in the world (which for AESOPs will be never!) you can put the photos in albums and catalogue the keepsakes. Better yet, you may have offspring who are compulsively neat, and you can simply pass the carefully labeled

> "Never decide to do nothing just because you can only do a little. Do what you can."
> -*Life's Little Treasure Book On Wisdom*

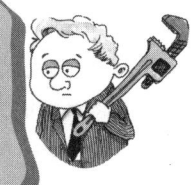

boxes off to them for arranging. No need for guilt here. You have managed to keep everything that is important. It even looks as though you have a carefully devised plan, even though you (and we) know it is really a carefully devised coping strategy.

Use the six month rule:

Everything is precious. It is painful to let go of anything you have accumulated, especially things that have held special meaning for you. Besides, in the past, just as soon as you have thrown something out, you invariably need it the next day or the next week. Try this: get a number of boxes with lids. Into these boxes place items that you THINK you can dispose of or that you won't need. Index the contents by writing on the box or use a 3x5 card to list the contents.

Seal the box and mark the date. Calculate a date, say either six or nine months in the future, and write this second date on the box in large red letters. Mark your calendar for that future date with "check box." If you have not needed to unseal the box to retrieve an item by the identified date, it is 99% certain that you truly can let go of that particular box. Have preset charities or disposal sites in mind. Dispose of the box without breaking the seal! This is important! If you unseal the box and look inside, the emotional tug will still be there.

Understand Feng Shui:

Feng Shui is an ancient Chinese art that places great significance on items and their location in the home. Practicing Feng Shui reduces clutter and increases serenity. We have our own version: we call it our quick and easy Feng Shui for AESOPs. Here is a list of questions you can ask yourself to help you deal with clutter in your home or office.

●Does my clutter impact anyone else? If your partner objects to stacks of papers, books, and magazines in the family room, consider screening that area off.

● Can I store these items? Decide whether some of your stacks are "storable." Can you operate without these things always at hand?

● Is it important as a family treasure? Wedding invitations and birth announcements are priceless family mementos. Do you have a special box or system ready for these?

● Is it safe? Protect papers against silverfish and excessive heat or dampness.

● Is it accessible? Have a labeling system that allows you to find what you've stored.

● Have I marked each box that I might get rid of with a "disposal deadline" and location for recycling or donation?

● Can I pare down the amount of paper? Remember to save single items, not whole newspapers to be read.

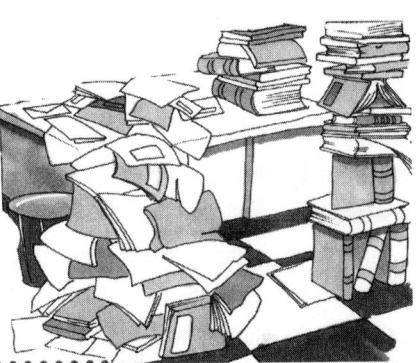

Protect yourself from a poor memory:

> "Cleaning your house when your kids are still growing is like shoveling the walk before it stops snowing."
> -*Phyllis Diller*

"Where did I put that?" is certainly a familiar AESOP lament. Use the idea of cross-referencing. On the box of 1992 photos, put a note that also references you to the other 1992 box marked "Schoolwork and Mementos" and vice versa.

Assess the consequences:

Are you about to hurt someone's feelings? If you have thank you notes to write from a year ago, or even more crucial, a sympathy card that needs to be sent, you need a plan of action which may include a person who will write them for you.

Hire a professional organizer:

If the piles continue to grow despite your best efforts, consider hiring a professional organizer who understands AESOPs. This person will come into your home and help you organize the immediate clutter, and more importantly, help you develop easy-to-use systems for clutter containment and management.

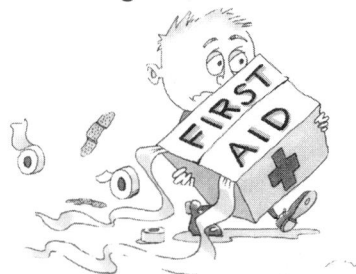

Need More First Aid?

If you feel like you can't even get started on the clutter because there's just too much, see:
Overwhelm in Chapter 1.

If your clutter leaves you feeling blue and unmotivated, see:
Depression in Chapter 17.

If you keep putting off tackling even the smallest part of your clutter, see:
Procrastination in Chapter 4.

AESOP=Adults Experiencing Special Operating Problems

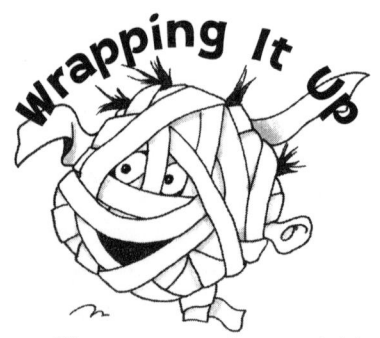

Wrapping It Up

- Clutter accumulates quickly and can overwhelm you.

- Working towards containment of clutter is more effective than thinking you'll be able to change your basic personality.

- You can use specific techniques and tools to start containing your clutter, including clumping, sorting, and dating.

- Clutter is a reality for many SOP Adults and will clamor for your attention on a regular basis.

> "Being a clutterer is a genetic trait. It will stick with you like Velcro, so don't plan to erase the tendency from your personality profile. After all, antique shops, museums, and archives all over the world exist because of people like you!"
>
> *-Joan and Denise*

AESOP=Adults Experiencing Special Operating Problems

Consistency

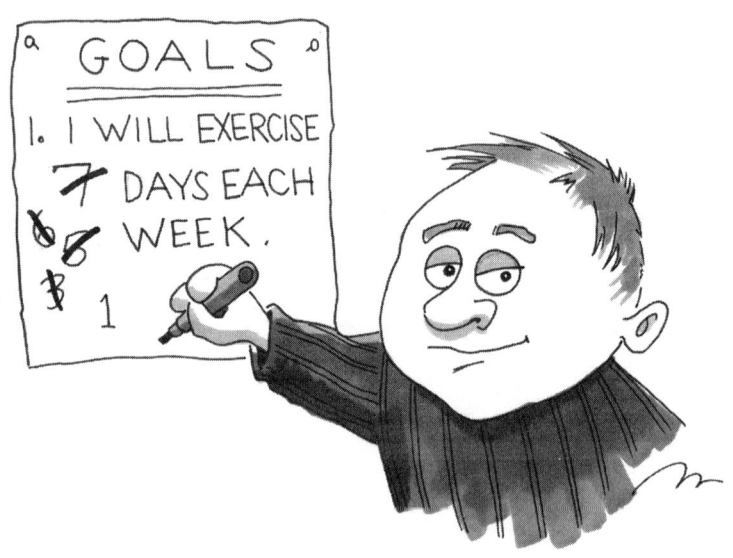

Chapter 8

What You Need To Know

Adults with SOP can be consistently inconsistent. With our unique body chemistries, we can expect periods of peak performance, offset by periods of immobility.

This tends to drive us (and others who don't understand) crazy, especially when we compare ourselves to other adults without special operating problems who seem to be moving through their lives at a consistent, steady pace. We find ourselves asking, "What's wrong with me? Why can't I diet, exercise, or stick to a schedule at work like everyone else?" Often, these questions lead to painful self-recriminations and a fear that we are lacking in drive or are truly lazy.

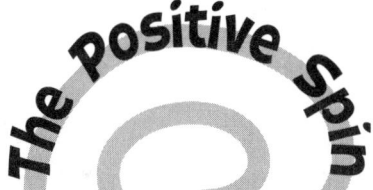

The Positive Spin

Instead of seeing "inconsistency" as a negative, realize there is an upside to this. With planning and the use of coping

AESOP=Adults Experiencing Special Operating Problems

> "If you have made mistakes...there is always another chance for you...you may have a fresh start any moment you choose, for this thing we call "failure" is not the falling down, but the staying down."
>
> *-Mary Pickford*

strategies, periods of peak performance can yield brilliance. These periods need to be recognized and prized. This in turn allows you to view your periods of immobility as relaxation and preparation for the next spurt, rather than feeling guilty that your body chemistry is in an "off" cycle.

Techniques
Recognize Your Rhythm:

Evaluate your best times of day or night or the time of year when you are most likely to pull off something big. Plan around those times as periods of probable peak performance. For example, if the Fall is a gloomy time for you, target Spring as the season to commit to that big project at work or to paint the house. If your peak times seem inconsistent, try to locate some pattern. Ask yourself, "Am I better at night or in the morning? At the beginning or end of the week?"

Isolate Parts:

Break projects into smaller, separate parts so that the completion of each part can coincide with one of your peak periods. Reward yourself as you complete a part in order to encourage yourself to keep working towards the whole. When all the pieces are finished and brought together, acknowledge that the project is complete. Praise yourself for a job well done, and give yourself permission to take that mini-vacation and embrace your downtime.

Looking productive at work:

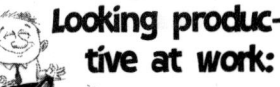

Even though you understand your unique pacing, your boss might not. Save mindless tasks such as stapling, three-hole punching, and straightening your desk

> "In the confrontation between the stream and the rock, the stream always wins--not through strength but by perseverance."
>
> -Dad

Feeling productive at home:

No boss to worry about here, just your own feelings about how productive you are on a daily basis. Plan larger projects such as Spring cleaning, painting baseboards, or washing rugs just as though you were in a work environment and tackling a big project. Fill in your periods of down-time with short-term tasks such as folding laundry or doing dishes. Establish a specific goal, whether it is making the surface of the house look neat or organizing that impossible storage closet. Once you have accomplished that goal, don't hesitate to curl up with a good book for some well earned downtime.

> "You must do the thing you think you cannot do."
> -Eleanor Roosevelt

Protect yourself from the "down days":

If you bottom out with depression and can't remember even simple tasks you planned to do, protect yourself. Start a list of the routine tasks that you thought of during your periods of peak performance but didn't want to waste creative energy doing at that time. Then you will have this list to mindlessly follow when you are in the dumps. In fact, doing something, anything at all, can often help us come out of a depressive slump.

Added tips to stay on track at home:

Regularly schedule routine tasks such as dry cleaning drop-off or laundry day on your calendar.

Use a timer to limit wasted time. Decide to dedicate fifteen minutes to cleaning up the kitchen, then set the timer. Working against the clock can be a stimulating challenge!

Use a third party:

There are tasks that need to

be done consistently and steadily such as paying bills, sending out birthday cards, doing deep house cleaning, etc. If, hard as you've tried, you haven't been able to stay on top of them, you may need to hire someone as the last, best resort. Sometimes hiring that third party on a regular basis generates consistency, i.e., many people clean up before the cleaning people arrive every other week, just to avoid the embarrassment!

> *"Progress is sometimes followed by a comma, never by a period."*
> -20,000 Quotes

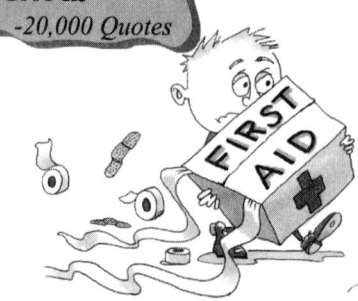

Need More First Aid?

If putting off a plan or goal is a problem, see:
Procrastination in Chapter 6.

If being easily distracted from your task or goal is a problem, see: **Distractibility in Chapter 10.**

> *"Periods of peak performance can yield brilliance."*
> —Joan and Denise

dictates when we're operating at peak performance or barely able to cope.

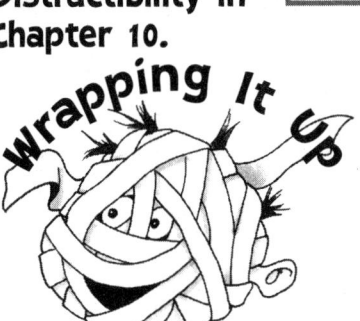

Wrapping It Up

- AESOPs often have difficulty remaining consistent in their tasks, plans, or goals.

- Body chemistry often dictates when we're operating at peak performance or barely able to cope.

- Identify your own personal cycles. Pay special attention to your peak periods and periods of immobility.

- Techniques are available to help you make the most of your peak times.

- We must also learn to be kinder to ourselves when we're "off peak."

Impulsivity

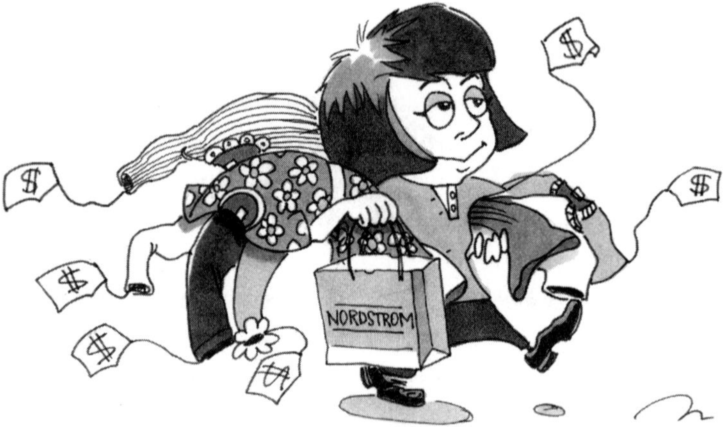

Chapter 9

What You Need To Know

"How did I get myself into this? I have a new car, a new VCR, but at the same time, I just walked off my job. I always do this to myself. It seems as if before I know what's happened, I've gotten myself into a pickle, not just once, but again and again." If you find yourself with questions like these, you are experiencing AESOP impulsivity.

The Positive Spin

Your marvelous brain with all its chemical impulses popping and flashing is awesome in its power. When you harness this power and provide direction to its intensity, you can accomplish anything! Yet unchecked, this same surge of electricity makes you move from one thing to another and can occasionally, or frequently, (or for some of us, inevitably) lead to rash decisions. Remember, with any powerful

AESOP = Adults Experiencing Special Operating Problems

force, we need to be able to set limits. Think in terms of harnessing this power. This requires providing direction to its intensity as well as enforcing a stopping point.

Looking back at your life, you may see patterns of impulsive spending, or sudden moves from one college, or one job, or one relationship to another. This is not a character flaw! This is your brain chemistry at work. Once you identify this pattern in yourself, you can successfully put fail-safe systems and controls in place.

Techniques
With Your Finances

Empty your wallet or purse of credit cards and checkbooks:

When you are shopping, the time it takes to go and retrieve a credit card before making a purchase can allow your impulsivity to settle. This lets you better assess, "Do I really need this?"

Use the 24-hour rule:

First, set a reasonable limit for your own income level,

> "Experience has taught me this; that we undo ourselves with impatience."
> -*Michel De Montaigne*

say $50, $100, or $1000. Then if the purchase is over that amount, make a promise to yourself that you will let 24 hours elapse before you go ahead with it.

Resist acting on the excitement of the moment:

If you quickly become caught up in the excitement of a venture that promises to make you an instant millionaire, slow yourself down. This is the time to reach out to trusted mentors, someone older and wiser in financial matters. Make a phone call and ask for their advice. If you disagree with them, promise to wait 48 hours, not just 24, before making a final decision.

Consider the pitfalls:

If the excitement of making big money, or of buying or selling gold, silver, or stocks is too enticing, stop for a moment. Sit down and calculate what will happen to your savings, nest egg, or retirement fund if, heaven forbid, you are wrong, and you lose all your investment. Then ask yourself: is the risk worth it?

Put on the brakes:

Do you have a tendency to move into excited phases of your life (almost manic in quality) where you lose sight of reality? During these times do you spend money to the detriment of your business or relationship? If so, make sure your mentor (or spouse) is aware and can help you identify when you are in this phase. Once you are fully engaged in this level of excitement, trust us, you will not be able to see the big picture yourself and will need another's objective point of view to stay out of trouble.

> "There's a lot we can do in the fast lane--we can grow and we can expand. But we cannot integrate our experiences unless we slow down."
> *-Angeles Arrien*

Chapter 9 • Impulsivity

Enlist the help of your partner or mentor:

If your spending is totally out of control, here is a drastic but effective solution. (Search for a rational moment when you are more in control and willing to take this step.) Enlist the help of your partner or mentor and arrange your checking account so that you will need two signatures on your checks.

Use the envelope system:

Each week, put money for food, entertainment, gas, etc., in labeled, separate envelopes. This way, you will be able to see the money disappear as you spend it. A thinning envelope lets you see that you're actually spending your money. It's much more immediate than swiping that little piece of plastic through the magnetic reader.

Find a professional life-preserver:

If all else fails, hire an accountant. Have your paycheck sent to that person who will pay your bills, make your investments, and give you an allowance. This is the most severe form of damage control but, at times, is very necessary.

In Your Relationships

Recognize the phases of love:

The first bloom and excitement of love is thrilling and wonderful. In a long-standing relationship, this inevitably settles down to a warm glow with occasional sparks. If you perceive this pattern as boring and wonder if you are falling out of love, hold your horses! Recognize this for what it is, a natural maturing process that occurs in every relationship.

Check your mating preferences:

When mate-hunting, take into account your own need for excitement and activity. If you love white-water rafting and mountain climbing, you may not be compatible with a spouse who loves to read and knit.

Preserve your relationship:

If you are already married or in a partnership with some-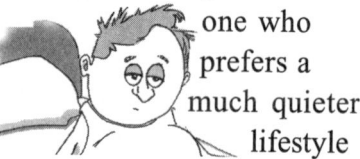one who prefers a much quieter lifestyle than you, know that in this case your stimulation must come from your own activities outside the home. You may need to provide time for soccer games with friends or mountain bike with a group or by yourself. You may even need to throw in an occasional bungee-jumping excursion. With enough stimulation in place to satisfy your own needs, you can work on seeing your home as a refuge, a place of safety and relaxation, rather than a place of boredom and confinement.

> "Remember this statement by Coach Lou Holtz, 'Life is 10 percent what happens to me and 90 percent how I react to it.'"
> —*Life's Little Treasure Book on Wisdom*

On the Job

Ask yourself: Are you truly in the wrong job?

Take a careful look at your job description or job requirements. If the job is truly boring or too routine, a

> "Who begins too much accomplishes little."
> *German Proverb*

carefully calculated job change might be the ticket.

Avoid frequent job changes:

If your past history is to remain in a job for only a year or so, recognize that this is your "boredom point." See this pattern for what it is and plan ahead for the inevitable by developing an exciting project at work, changing work locations, or taking an adventurous vacation to break the monotony.

Seek socially acceptable job changes:

Investigate the possibility of changing jobs or territories within the same company. Possibly a move to Alaska or Timbuktu will change the way you feel about your job, even though you might be doing the same routine tasks.

Learn to cope with tedium:

If paperwork, reports, or expense accounts are a required part of your job, understand that tackling them will feel tedious and overwhelming. Know that your resistance to these feelings may make you want to bolt from the scene and plan ways to reduce the tedium by improving your systems of paperwork. In extreme situations, consider hiring someone to complete the nitty-gritty paper and pencil minutia for you.

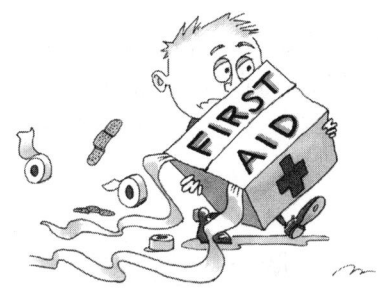

Need More First Aid?

If handling money provokes your impulsivity, see:
Money in Chapter 12.

For more information on relationships in general, see:
Help for Yourself in a Relationship, in

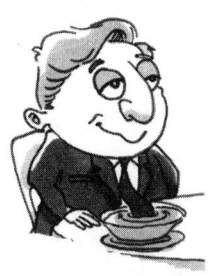

Chapter 21, and Help for Your Partner and Family in a Relationship in Chapter 22.

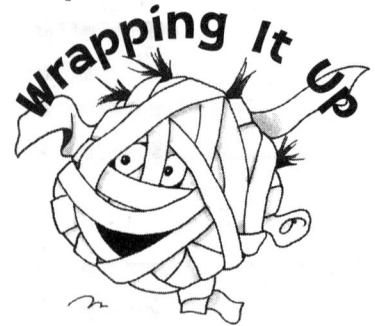

Wrapping It Up

- Impulsivity often creates havoc for AESOPs and can impact how money is handled and how success in a career or a relationship is achieved.

- AESOPs' specialized brain chemistry is the culprit in this case, and it can lead to snap decisions that may have disastrous consequences.

- Once the pattern of impulsivity is identified, there are techniques that will allow you to get things under control.

- Realistically, life-long control of impulsivity requires vigilance as well as long-range planning.

> "Your marvelous brain with all its chemical impulses popping and flashing is awesome in its power. When you harness this power and provide direction to its intensity, you can accomplish anything!"
>
> *-Joan and Denise*

Distractibility

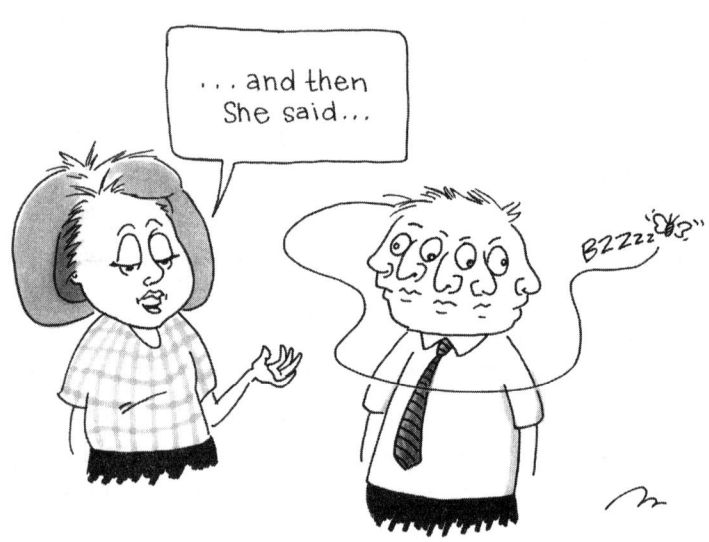

Chapter 10

What You Need To Know

Do you feel scattered? Do you find yourself paying attention to several things at once, although to none of them very well? Staying on track and screening out all the stimulation around us is really difficult for Adults with SOP. Distractibility is increased with stress, and our attention span can feel like soap that slips out of our hands and is picked up only to quickly slip out of our hands once more. This can be incredibly frustrating for ourselves and for those around us.

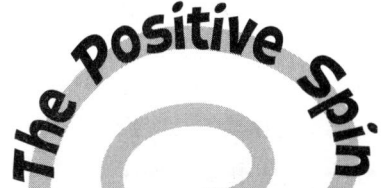

The Positive Spin

There are days when you can focus and days when you can't, no matter how hard you try. On good days, which are unfortunately impossible to predict, you can focus clearly. These days provide precious opportunities to dive in and solve some of the more pressing distractions themselves, such as the clutter of paperwork

AESOP=Adults Experiencing Special Operating Problems

around you or the fact that there is no clear path leading from the kitchen to your bedroom. For the not-so-good days, learn to recognize the conditions that distract you. Be gentle with yourself if your distractibility is out of control. Develop a repertoire of coping techniques that will get you through those times with as much grace as possible. For example, in an office or at a restaurant, don't sit facing the door so that every passerby catches your eye. Instead, choose a chair that faces a wall so that your only choices are to pay attention to the person you're talking to or to the blank wall itself.

Techniques

Use peak time:

Evaluate your best times of day or night, or the best time of year, (when are you most likely to pull off something big or complicated?) and plan on using those times as periods of optimum performance. For example, if the Fall is a gloomy time for you, target Spring to commit to that big project at work or to paint the house. If ten o'clock at night is your peak time, tackle your most complex task then, not at six in the morning.

> "Learn to recognize the inconsequential; then ignore it." -Life's Little Treasure Book On Wisdom

Narrow your focus:

Break projects into smaller, separate parts so that completion of each part can take place during one of your peak periods. Reward yourself as you complete each; this will provide the encouragement to keep going. (If you find you've gotten lost, you may have moved out of your peak time; try using timers or lists to help you retain your focus.)

When the pieces are finished and brought together, acknowledge that the project is completed. Praise yourself for a job well done, and then give yourself permission to take that mini-vacation. And remember to embrace your relaxation time!

Restrict your environment:

Adults with SOP tend to fall into two categories: those who need absolute silence to focus and concentrate and those who must have background noise. If you fall into the first category, turn off the TV, turn off your pager and cell phone, and eliminate all background noises. If you fall into the second category, introduce background noise that helps you narrow your focus and reduces distractibility: try music, white noise, or even talk radio.

> "The road to success has many tempting parking places."
> -Steve Potter

Control for boredom:

Distractibility at home or at work may be caused by routine tasks that are so boring that you'd do anything to escape them. If this is the case, try using a timer, working to a deadline, or setting small rewards for yourself at the completion of each task.

Contain wandering thoughts:

Whether you are distracted by worry or by the excitement of a new adventure, you may find those particular thoughts replaying constantly in your mind. Consider two approaches: The first is to examine the thought that is causing the distractibility and actively solve the problem. If this is not possible, the other approach is to give yourself permission to think about it for a specific amount of time. Attend to the distraction, and then make an agreement with yourself to move on.

Keep a distraction list handy:

If random thoughts about sending a thank you note, picking up milk on the way home, or filling in the hole the dog dug in the yard keep cropping up in your mind, keep a blank piece of paper or notepad close by to jot down your distractions. Once you've jotted them down, tell yourself to let them go. This reduces the clutter in your mind, and also insures that you won't forget the important minutia.

Where that distraction list goes depends on whether it contains "to do" action items or just worry thoughts that don't require further action.

Monitor your medication:

One of the biggest complaints of AESOPs is their

distractibility. Remember that some medications may directly *improve* your ability to focus and thereby *reduce* your distractibility. There is often a double-bind wherein the worry over whether to medicate or not can be a distraction in itself! Counting out your pills in the morning or keeping them in a seven-day pillbox can help.

Put your best foot forward:

Even though you understand your unique pacing, your boss might not. Save mindless tasks such as stapling, three-hole punching, or straightening your desk for those times when you are recovering from your peak period so that you'll still look busy and be accomplishing something, albeit minor.

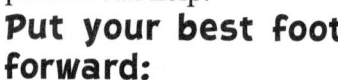

"When you can't solve the problem, manage it."
-*Robert H. Schuller*

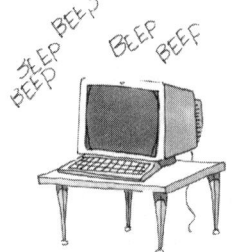

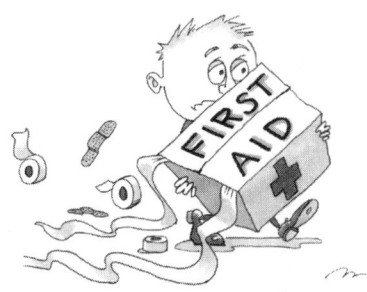

Need More First Aid?

If you have too much on your plate and are not only stressed but totally overloaded, check out:
Chapter 1 on Overwhelm and Chapter 2 on Stress Reduction.

If you need more help in seeking solutions for your distractibility, see:
Problem-Solving in Chapter 3.

If you have problems using and organizing your time wisely, see:
Organization in Chapter 4 and/or Time Management in Chapter 5.

AESOP=Adults Experiencing Special Operating Problems

Wrapping It Up

- Identify your very best time of day or of the year and plan to tackle a big project with your optimum performance period in mind.

- Some days will inevitably be worse than others when it comes to distractibility.

> "Be like a postage stamp. Stick to something until you get there." -Josh Billings

- Identify when you are having a bad day, and put specific coping techniques in place to minimize the problems.

- Your level of distractibility can be affected by your stress level. If you have too much on your plate at any one time, distractibility will increase.

- Don't ignore your distractibility or try to pretend

that it doesn't exist. Understand its roots and put coping techniques in place to minimize its effects on your life.

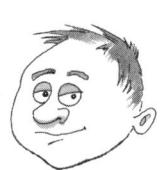

> "For the not-so-good days, learn to recognize the conditions that distract you. Be gentle with yourself if your distractibility is out of control. Develop a repertoire of coping techniques that will get you through those times with as much grace as possible."
>
> *-Joan and Denise*

Strategies for Death, Taxes and Other Necessary Evils

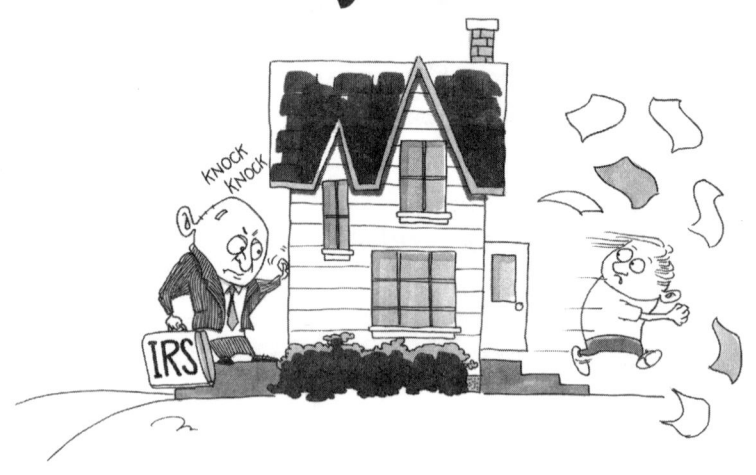

Chapter 11

What You Need To Know

There are things we have to do that are tedious and just plain boring. Many of these tasks trigger the AESOPs' avoidance behaviors. This section gives specific suggestions for some of those time-consuming, energy-draining tasks, such as paying bills, doing taxes, keeping a mileage log, writing important letters, and saving important documents.

This chapter includes tools and strategies for:

- Paying bills
- Dealing with creditors
- Preparing your taxes
- Keeping records
- Maintaining your life history
- Accessing work or school accommodations
- Plus specific ideas for accommodations at the University/College level

The Positive Spin

Though AESOPs may find these tasks a challenge, hav-

AESOP = Adults Experiencing Special Operating Problems

ing systems in place to tackle them efficiently can be a real boost to our sense of accomplishment, especially since we've struggled with them before. After all, life can be tough. With all the demands made on us, in fact life can be a real pain. In the new millennium, the best way to keep your head above water is to tackle each requirement of our civilization head-on.

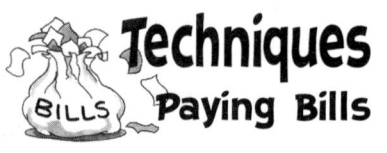

Techniques
Paying Bills

Put all incoming mail in one special place:

For example, put every piece of mail in a box or a basket until you sort it into junk mail, bills, correspondence. This way you don't lose anything.

Use a bill payment center:

When you do sort your mail, have one particular place for bills. Many office supply stores now have bill payment centers for just this purpose. They are rugged containers with places for envelopes, return address labels, stamps, incoming bills, and outgoing mail.

Chapter 11 • Death, Taxes...

There's a slot in the top where bills can be inserted as soon as you get them to eliminate the scattered bill syndrome. If you're not using a bill payment center, you need to designate a box or a container exclusively for bill paying.

Target one or two "bill" days a month:

Designate two days, i.e., the first and the 20th, for bill paying. Mark these days on your calendar or in your day-timer for months ahead until you get into a routine.

Set specific payment due dates:

If you pay property taxes, IRS estimates, or insurance premiums, mark those due dates for the entire year on your calendar or day-timer as soon as you get the bills. Because these particular bills are not your monthly regular bills, special attention must be given to calendar them.

Use a clumping technique:

Items need to be centralized in one place. This will eliminate going off on tangents as you search for something that is out of place. In the bill payment center example, the idea is to have your bills, stamps, return labels, and checks all in one place. Another example would be to have your gloves, clippers, rose food, and garbage bags in one place for pruning time. If you do this, when you're ready to take action you won't have to jump up every few minutes to get something you forgot and run the risk of being further distracted from your goal.

Consider automatic payment plans:

Many utility and mortgage companies have automatic payment plans that deduct the billed amount directly from your bank account. If you use this method, you must remember to deduct the amount from your balance in the check register.

Dealing with Creditors

Write letters to your creditors:

Many AESOPs have trouble paying bills (or even finding them). We often feel angry or embarrassed as the late notices come in and tend to avoid our creditors even more. It's possible

Chapter 11 • Death, Taxes...

that your creditors will quiet down if you contact them with a payment proposal. Here is a sample letter:

Big Department Store
555 W. Fifth Street
Anywhere, Any State Zip

Re: Your Account Number
To Whom It May Concern:

I am writing to request a payment plan be set up between us so that I can meet my obligations to you in a reasonable way.

I currently owe $_____ and, as a show of good faith, would like to pay $_____ each month toward that bill. Please notify me as soon as possible with your decision. Thank you for your consideration of my request.

Sincerely,

(Your signature)

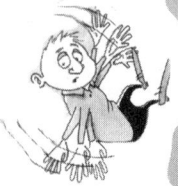

> "Every great mistake has a halfway moment, a split second when it can be recalled and perhaps remedied."
> -Pearl S. Buck

Consider consulting a consumer credit bureau:

Many states now have consumer agencies that can matter-of-factly look at your bills, indebtedness, and overall financial picture. These services are usually low cost and very practical about what your options are. They are usually located in the phone book under Credit.

Preparing Your Taxes

Keep all receipts for the same year together:

This is especially tricky in the December of the past year to January of the new year changeover, but is very important.

Use accordion files:

In these files, stash away your tax stuff. If the labeled categories don't fit your situation, make your own category labels and stick them over the top. If "Auto" doesn't click immediately for you, re-label it "Car," so it's user friendly.

Use a checking account program on the computer:

There are many programs available for the computer that will help by tracking finances electronically. Have them demonstrated before you buy one. It must be easy for you to use, or it'll just be one more piece of software you didn't need.

Use a tax program if you file your own taxes:

Many of today's computerized tax programs scout out red flags and math errors. These can be a godsend for an AESOP.

Use a financial planner and/or a tax consultant:

If any of your circumstances seem questionable, don't be afraid to seek professional advice. A tax audit is an AESOP's nightmare. ("You want me to locate records from which year?") Don't set yourself up for trouble; get help from an expert. Incidentally, this can be helpful even if your circumstances don't seem questionable! Having someone else go over your paperwork and figures--and promising to be there in case of an audit--is a great mental relief for some of us, even if our taxes are simple.

Use a mileage log:

You can save a ton of money on your taxes if you have a system of charting mileage and keep it simple. Consider using a mileage log that can track beginning and ending mileage each day. Check with your accountant or tax planner to confirm which mileage is allowable. Above all, don't count on your memory!

What You Need to Keep

Save your warranties and instruction manuals:

Write the date and place of purchase on the front of each warranty. Keeping these helps avoid huge service fees if your machine is still covered under warranty when it glitches. It also allows you to order the proper parts if something breaks. Warranties should be kept in a separate, permanent accordion file, not your yearly tax file.

Keep all tax records:

According to the Internal Revenue Service's Policies and Procedures Department, you must keep all of your receipts and records for three years if you are an individual and seven years if you are a business owner. After taxes are filed for that year, your records should be bundled and stored safely and accessibly along with your check registers and appointment book, in case of an audit.

TAX ALERT:

If you have ever had tax problems such as an audit, even if it was a favorable audit, you will be set up for further scrutiny. Make sure you keep tax records for that year. If the audit was negative as an individual or business owner, the IRS states that you must keep your records for all years FOREVER.

Protect your automobile documents:

Keep the pink slip in your safe deposit box, a home safe, or a lock box, and your car loan documents, repair records and warranties in your accordion file. Keep your car registration and insurance receipts in the glove box. You can save money, time, and sometimes a ticket if you can get your hands on these easily.

Retain your immunization records:

Keep these in your permanent accordion file or safe deposit box for yourself and your family in the event of booster shots, an emergency, a copy requested by the school, or plans to enter a country with vaccination requirements.

Guard your passports:

A passport is valid for ten years. Applying for one can be a pain because of all the original documents requested (no copies allowed). Keep it safe!

Maintaining a History of Your Life

None of us likes to think in terms of retirement, old age, or even worse, death. However, as the old saying goes, death and taxes are inevitable; paying attention to this category will save you and your loved ones from delay and aggravation.

The following list of items

are all crucial over the course of your life. If you can reach into a drawer when you are 65 ton of money in taxes.

These items should be kept in a home safe or in a safe

> "The secret of getting ahead is getting started. The secret of getting started is breaking your complex overwhelming tasks into small manageable tasks, and then starting on the first one."
>
> -*Mark Twain*

or 70 and miraculously emerge with these vital documents you will save yourself hours of time and energy researching things such as "Just how much did I pay for my first house in 1954?" and also a deposit box. Be sure at least one other member of the family knows where these records are kept and has access to them. This means that they will not only need to know the location of the safe deposit key, but also have their name on the signature card for access, or they will need keys/combination to the house safe or lock box.

Birth certificate(s):

You can request your original Birth Certificate (if you don't already have it) by contacting the county where you were born. This is not something we usually remember to set safely aside (or even think about). Get it now to avoid stress in the future when you want to get a passport, prove citizenship, etc.

Original social security card(s):

There are circumstances (although rare) when the same social security number is issued to more than one person in error. Keep your and your family's original cards safe.

Comprehensive list of bank accounts:

Compile a list of all of your checking accounts, savings accounts and account numbers of money held by any financial institutions. This list should be on record both for you to track your assets and liabilities and in the event of an emergency.

Stocks and bonds:

Keep a record of the original purchase price of all stocks and bonds (with canceled checks if applicable). These will be necessary for tax purposes if you decide to sell them to prove the amount of profit or loss.

Life insurance papers:

Keep a list of your policies and coverage amounts; these will be necessary in the event of an emergency, or if you are permitted to take a loan against the face value.

Wills and trusts:

First, be sure you have a will! Second, be aware that wills and trusts will need to be updated if you add property, buy a new house, or change any designees. If trusts are not revised, there will be a substantial loss of income for your family at your death as your estate will need to go through probate. No matter how young and healthy you are, no matter whether it's personally or professionally prepared, you should have a will and/or trust. (You can prepare your own holographic will, but your trust must be done by an attorney.)

> *"Anxiety is the interest paid on trouble before it is due."*
> -William Inge

House title deeds:

Keep every single piece of paper that directly relates to each house you have ever owned. You will need proof of the original purchase price, and receipts for home improvements such as new carpeting, a new fence, a remodeled bathroom. You'll also need proof of any loses you in-incurred due to fire or earthquake (especially if they were not covered by insurance). This sounds like a huge task, but it will pay off big time in saving you tax money at retirement or upon the sale of your home.

Capital gains:

Save receipts and canceled checks that can be used to adjust your original purchase price and reduce your capital gains. Again, this will save you tax dollars at retirement or sale of the property.

Accessing Work or School Accommodations

Decide whether to tackle work or school problems alone or with help:

Identify the types of work problems you're having. As you brainstorm possible solutions, pay attention to your thoughts and feelings. Are you too overwhelmed? Are your thoughts too scattered in order for you to come up with solutions? Do you have trusted resource people who can help?

Familiarize yourself with the Americans with Disabilities Act (ADA):

Special Note: If you are an AESOP who has been identified with a learning disability, Attention Deficit Disorder, or a physical disability, you may be able to request accommodations at work or at school.

The Americans with Disabilities Act (ADA) has specific, narrow criteria you must meet in order to be protected by the ADA, and therefore, eligible for accommodations. These criteria include: physical or mental conditions which impair one or more major life activities and/or having a record of such impairment. To qualify, a diagnosis must be made by an appropriate licensed professional and verified on paper.

This act is very specific in its mandate that disabled workers are entitled to reasonable accommodations in order to perform their jobs. A sample list of accommodations follows:

- less distracting work environment
- modified work hours
- extended time on any and all tests given before and during employment or school matriculation.
- in the workplace, restructuring the job, i.e. reviewing job descriptions and modifying tasks when appropriate

Contact ADA resource numbers:

For quick information about the ADA, call:

Job Accommodation Network
(800)232-9675

U.S. Department of Justice
Civil Rights Division

Disability Rights Section
ADA Information Line
(800) 514-0301
www.usdoj.gov

What if I don't qualify under the ADA and still need special accommodations in my workplace?

The emphasis in the American workplace is on productivity. Everyone has their strengths and weaknesses, not just AESOPs. If you offer a sound proposal to your employer, with very concrete solutions, he or she may be willing to accommodate you without you having to invoke a law. An example might be approaching your employer about having specific blocks of time to return phone calls and other blocks of time dedicated to paperwork. Point out that this proposal would help you boost productivity since you would not be continually distracted, bouncing between phone and papers.

Accessing Accommodations at the University or College Level

Get help when applying: Many colleges have a special admission procedure for certain AESOPs. If you have an identified learning or physical disability, you may be accommodated differently to better address your pattern of disability. Prior to applying for admission, it's a good idea to visit the campus and drop in on the Disabled Student Center. Be prepared to assess for yourself whether this school will provide a helpful environment for you.

Sometimes standardized entrance exams can also be accommodated:

You may be entitled to a distraction-free testing environment, extended time, the use of a computer, or a reader. Again the criteria for eligibility is strict, so use your designated school administrator or counselor for help.

"Yes, I'm eligible":

The campus you attend can use a letter such as the sample on the following page to request accommodations and services once you have been identified as an AESOP who is entitled to accommodations.

Special note:

The following are accommodations that are typically

requested:
- Student needs to read test information aloud in order to process information.
- Student needs to use computer for essay tests.
- Student needs permission to tape record lectures.
- Student requires use of calculator during tests.
- Student requires extended time to take tests.
- Student requires alternative location to take exams (usually the Learning Disability Center).
- Student needs to use an alternative test method to scantron testing.

Use campus resources:

Whether your SOP is clearly identified or just becoming noticeable to you, there are many resources on campus to provide help, support, and possible modifications.

Examples of these services are: Tutoring Centers, Learning Disability Programs, Disabled Student Services, Counseling Services.

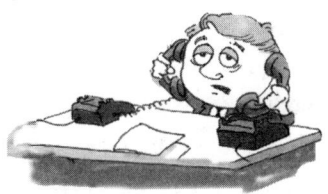

```
WE CARE UNIVERSITY
Date:
To:      PROFESSOR'S NAME, SUBJECT
From:    DISABLED STUDENT CENTER STAFF OR COUNSELOR
RE:      NAME OF STUDENT AND I.D. NUMBER
```

(Name) was referred to the Disabled Student Center this semester with documentation that he/she has _____ (accepted SOP title goes here).

Because of his/her learning difficulties, he/she may need special accommodations to insure improved performance. (Name) is having difficulty with the time constraints of testing situations and would benefit from an alternative test site with extended time.

We will be happy to assist you in arranging for these accommodations. Please feel free to contact us at 555-5555 regarding any questions you may have.

Signature of
Counselor_____

Date_____

Chapter 11 • Death, Taxes...

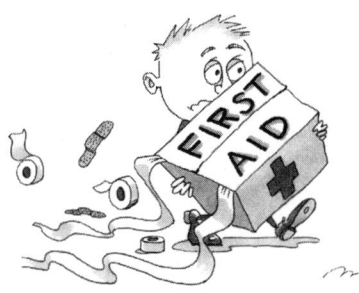

Need More First Aid?

If clutter is a problem in keeping bills, permanent records, correspondence, and magazine articles separated, see:
Clutter in Chapter 7.

If you have trouble with finances and managing money, see:
Money in Chapter 12.

If you're having trouble at work and aren't sure how to sort it out before requesting accommodations, see:
Problems at Work in Chapter 25.

If you want more information on the kinds of problems that might crop up in school before you request accommodations, see:
Problems in School in Chapter 27.

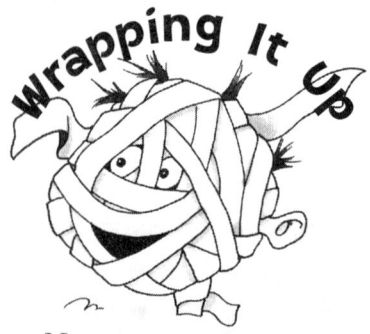

Wrapping It Up

- No matter who we are, there will always be bills to pay, records to keep and paperwork to do.

- There are tools and tips available for paying bills, dealing with creditors, keeping and filing taxes, and record-keeping.

- Sometimes, keeping yourself out of trouble might require work or school accommodations--formal or informal.

- Colleges and universities can often provide accommodations to help you better master higher education.

- Keeping yourself out of trouble can be managed with tools and techniques. By staying with it, you won't get buried under the paperwork.

Chapter 11 • Death, Taxes...

> "With all the demands made on us, life can be a real pain. The best way to keep your head above water is to tackle each requirement of our civilization head-on."
>
> -Joan and Denise

Money

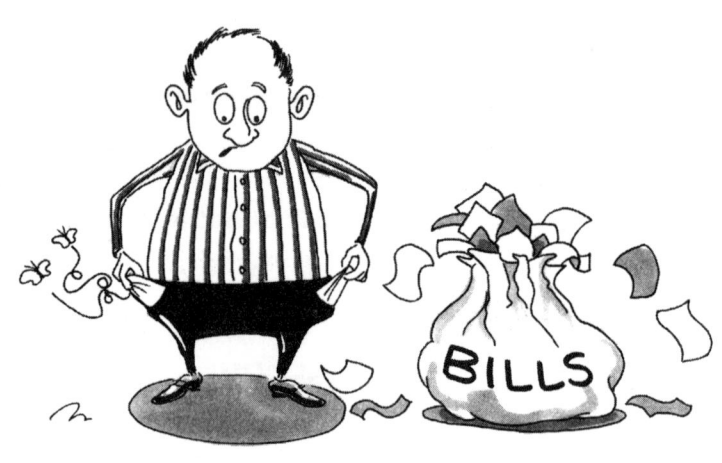

Chapter 12

What You Need To Know

Money problems come from the inability to regulate on a daily basis how much money goes out of your hands. It is also the inability to conceptualize future needs such as taxes, a balloon payment on a house, or insurance. Problems exist whether someone has a steady paycheck coming in, whether they get paid in lump sums that fluctuate in amount and timing, or whether there isn't much money coming in at all.

The Positive Spin

Acknowledge to yourself that while managing money is doable, it is certainly a pain in the neck and not nearly as much fun as riding the edge and feeling the excitement of spending. Nevertheless, managing money is one of those things that we must do because if we don't, the possible consequences are disastrous. Having to face bankruptcy, the IRS knocking at your door,

AESOP=Adults Experiencing Special Operating Problems

the electricity and phones being shut off are examples.

Techniques
Spending

Note: The following techniques are presented from least restrictive to most restrictive. Choose the appropriate level depending on your level of difficulty.

Create a bill paying center:

Stamps, pens, return address labels, and bills must be all in one place. Some office supply stores actually sell ready-made bill paying centers.

Use envelopes:

These can be used in two ways for money management. First, cash your salary check (this system will work whether you are paid weekly, bimonthly or monthly). Label separate envelopes by category, such as food, electric bill, gas bill, etc. Put cash into the individual envelopes. Visually this will allow you to know when you are close to exceeding your limit. If a bill is to be paid once a month, such as the electric bill, convert the cash accumulated in the "electric bill envelope" into a money order once a month and send it off.

> "No one ever went broke saving money."
> -Dad

Use checking and saving sub-accounts:

Many banks will allow you to set up a Christmas account or a vacation account within your main account that can't be touched without a teller override. These can be set up for voluntary or automatic deposits.

Consider direct deposit of your paycheck:

This reduces the temptation of spending your money on the way to the bank and ensures that the deposit will be made in time.

Automatic payments:

Make arrangements with your bank to have enough money automatically deposited each month to pay off your regular ongoing bills: car payment, house payment, etc. Check with your utility company and other places that send you regular monthly bills. See if you can set up the same type of arrangement

> "Installment buying is popular because it enables you to live within your income as well as beyond your means." *-20,000 Quotes*

with them.

Leave your checkbook and credit cards at home:

This allows a time delay for you to rethink your purchase and let your rational self take over. If you can't conceptualize the big picture of how much money goes in and out, buy a dry erase board to track your expenses. List categories of money coming in, expenses going out, money in checking, money in savings, and larger expenses such as taxes.

Get help from a friend:

Target a rational, astute friend who manages money well and ask him or her to help you set up a financial system.

Get professional help:

Pay for an hour or two of your accountant or CPA's time to set up a feasible financial plan. Be sure to evaluate whether the methods or tools suggested will work for you and your type of SOP. If not, the plan won't be successful.

Turn over your entire check to your accountant or CPA:

Your expenses would then be managed from that location. You would receive an allowance for personal expenses.

Saving

Do you need savings? If so, what for? Be clear about your goal before you begin saving. It makes the process easier. Do you need money for retirement? Do you have kids and need a college fund, a remodel, money for a vacation or a house?

Do a reality check:

How much can you really afford to put into savings so that you don't have to touch it every time you fall short on the bills? To do this you must carefully analyze what's coming in and what's going out on both the short and long term. Again, consider getting help from a friend or a CPA with this analysis.

Start small with your savings:

Set yourself up so that you will succeed! Consider $5.00 a week or $20.00 a month at first.

Decide how you will save:

Choose whether you're going to save by physically putting money somewhere each week or month, or whether a direct deposit savings plan arranged by your bank with money going directly into savings without ever coming into your hands would be better for you.

> "The most popular labor-saving device is still money."
> -Phyllis George

Give yourself a six-month trial period, and then re-evaluate your plan:

If you didn't save at all before, and you managed to save four months out of six, recognize this as real improvement.

Chapter 12 • Money

Find out what plans are available through your work:

Some employers have programs that allow employees to set aside money for retirement using tax-deferred accounts. Some employers will also match a percentage of the employee's contribution. These are great opportunities. Check with the benefits person in your company's personnel office for details.

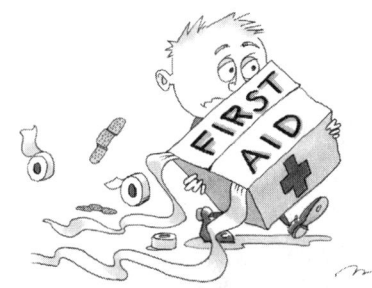

Need More First Aid?

If you find you are having trouble even identifying (much less solving) problems with money, see:

Problem Solving in Chapter 3.

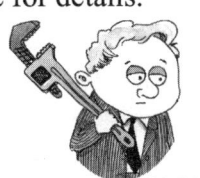

If you don't want to even

think about paying bills or if you kid yourself that other things are certainly more important in life, see:
Procrastination in Chapter 6.

If you can't seem to follow any plan for any length of time, see:
Consistency in Chapter 8.

If acting before thinking consistently gets you into trouble, see:
Impulsivity in Chapter 9.

> "Why is there so much month left at the end of the money?" -*Unknown*

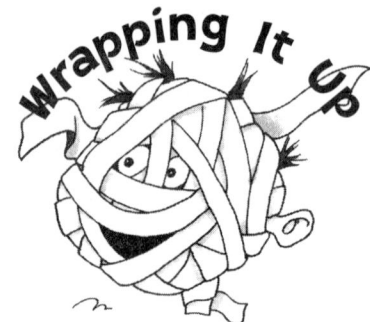

Wrapping It Up

- Money flows into our lives and can flow out of our lives much too quickly if we don't have a system to contain our expenditures.

Chapter 12 • Money

- Setting up techniques or routines to control our money is not nearly as much fun as the pure excitement of spending, but is very necessary to survive in our complicated world.

- Using very simple techniques can make a world of difference in our ability to save, control spending, and generally keep ourselves out of hot water.

> "Managing money is one of those things that we must do because if we don't, the possible consequences are disastrous."
>
> *-Joan and Denise*

Self-Sabotage

Chapter 13

What You Need To Know

Self-sabotage is a distinct and especially painful problem for AESOPs. It is a pattern of behavior that can't be explained fully by any one facet of our SOP. It goes beyond elements of depression that we may be dealing with. It goes beyond feeling anxious about our capabilities. Self-sabotage is a behavior (or lack of behavior) that seems so totally out of character and hard to understand, that it leaves an AESOP wondering "What in the world is the matter with me?".

Simply put, self-sabotage is like shooting yourself in the foot. It is the time that you have a birthday gift purchased, wrapped, and ready to mail, but you let it sit on the counter. Finally, the birthday is long past and you are too embarrassed to send the gift at all. The proposed recipient has no option but to feel that they have been forgotten. When you ask yourself, "Why did I do that?" you can come up with no answer. It is also the time when past hurts, like

AESOP=Adults Experiencing Special Operating Problems

hearing the high school counselor say, "Go to trade school, you'll never make it in college," swirl around and around in your head finally escalating to an all-consuming anger that makes you unable to think clearly or get anything done. You ask yourself "Why can't I let this go?" but you can come up with no answer.

For AESOPs, the entire subject of self-sabotage becomes a knotty problem. It is obvious that you are hitting some type of a roadblock. The question is, why? Because many AESOPs have co-occurring conditions (a little bit of depression, a little bit of anxiety, a little bit of anger, a little bit of this or that) you will need to take an additional step. You will need to tease out elements of any related conditions that may be presenting roadblocks on their own. Once that process occurs, you may have the ability to look clearly at the behavior and ask the important question "Am I doing this to myself?" Too often, we never ask that question.

Although at some level AESOPs are aware that we

are messing up an aspect of our lives, self-sabotage is usually the last possibility we can't do it."

For an Adult with SOP, self-sabotage typically comes in

> "Don't burn bridges. You'll be surprised at how many times you have to cross the same river."
> -*Life's Little Treasure Book On Wisdom*

consider. It is beyond our comprehension that we would be doing this to ourselves. The first clue that we are dealing with self-sabotage might be a sick feeling in the pit of our stomachs and thoughts that float through our minds such as: "I'm worthless; I'm stupid; I'll never learn; and I two forms. The first is not taking action when you know you should, such as with paying taxes, taking medication, paying your bills, or writing a thank you note. The other is holding onto negative thoughts and endlessly rehashing past failures such as poor grades in school, getting fired, or experiencing failures in relationships. Either of these types of self-sabotage can bring the adult to a despairing halt, physically and mentally.

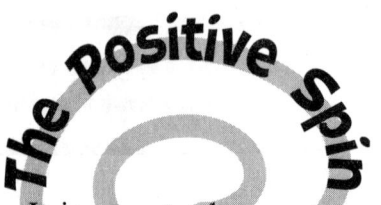
The Positive Spin

It is easy to throw up our hands and say "I'm helpless; I can't do it; it's not my fault." Come out of the victim position and realize that you have the ability to put yourself in control of your actions and your thoughts. It's a conscious choice. Empower yourself!

Recognizing why you may be stopping yourself and then facing that realization can be very empowering. Realize that you do have the ability to put yourself in control, even though you may have to repeat this process more than once. Make a conscious choice to empower yourself and then be prepared to remain vigilant!

Techniques
Break the problem into small pieces:

This will help you identify where the specific block

occurs. For example, if you don't pay your taxes, what's the real problem? Is your tax information scattered throughout three rooms? Are you worried you won't find it all--especially things like your W-2 which would be embarrassing to try to replace? Does reading the IRS booklet send you up the wall--or to the couch for a nap? Are you afraid of the math involved? Once you've identified the real problem, working it out becomes a specific task rather than an overwhelming specter of doom, which sets you up for self-sabotage.

Make a written list:

List the pros and cons of your task. Identify each stumbling block and be absolutely clear of the consequences if the task is not done.

> "We can always find something crazy to do in order for us to avoid doing what we know we should be doing."
> *-Melody Beattie*

For example, let's take the subject of something as simple as writing a thank-you note. The "pros" of writing it include: it would make you feel good about yourself and the thought of it hanging over your head would be put to rest. The "cons" of not writing it would be: you would feel badly about yourself, or you would beat yourself up for procrastination yet again. In a social situation, you would either avoid the person or blurt out an apology, you would feel generally guilty, and you would find yourself asking, "What in the world is the matter with me?"

This exercise certainly makes everything crystal clear, doesn't it?

Try the empty chair technique:

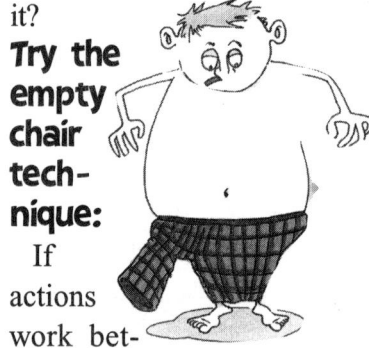

If actions work better for you than writing, try the following technique: choose one specific issue where you think you might be blocking yourself. Locate two chairs and place them facing each other; they will represent the two sides of the issue or argument. Think about the side you identify with more strongly. Sit in one chair to verbalize all your thoughts and opinions from that side. When you have run out of steam on that side, change chairs and speak strictly from the other side. A sample dialogue might relate to the task of returning daily phone calls. Side 1: "I absolutely hate to return phone calls. I talk all day. I don't want to get trapped on the phone. What I have to say can't be that important anyway." Change sides and become Side 2: "I have been sitting by the phone all day waiting for a call. I just need a minute of their time. I must not be important, or I'd get that call. I am so disappointed." The realization from this exchange might be that you see your call is very important to the other person and that they are counting on you. Your fear of not having anything important to say becomes clarified as part of your issue.

> "Never cut what can be untied."
> -Life's Little Treasure Book On Wisdom

Gradually the sides should unite to uncover what and why you're involved in self-sabotage.

Have a look at your priorities:

We often self-sabotage by doing a task that doesn't get us far as opposed to one that moves our lives forward. Calculate what the impact will be if you do one task over another. An example of a self-sabotaging priority would be getting a load of clothes washed rather than getting the bills mailed on time. Yes, the clothes do need washing, which may be an easier and less anxiety-producing activity, and still gives us a sense of being "on task" and productive; however, in the long run, putting off the bills will produce even more anxiety and have serious consequences.

Distinguish when self-sabotage is hidden:

When we hit a wall, an easy out is to target one of our SOPs and use it as an excuse. Are you addicted to television? Can't work without a nap first? Find yourself making three pleasure calls before

> "There's no power in victimhood. It isn't that you might not have had bad experiences, and it isn't that the pain is not real. But it's a loser's game to get stuck on 'Look what was done to me!' The only power is in 'Fine! It's all true. Now what am I going to do? What options exist for me?'"
>
> -Nathaniel Branden

making that important business call? You say to yourself, "Aha, I'm depressed. That is why I am having problems." The label of depression gives you an easy out. It may not be depression at all, but a form of self-sabotage. Sometimes, self-sabotage disguises itself as depression. While there may be co-occurring conditions, this form of depression may be caused by a response to negative thoughts and beliefs about not being able to move forward. Look around and see if you've developed any elaborate rituals that sabotage your progress.

Examine your fears and upsets for other origins of self-sabotage:

At times, self-sabotage is harder to identify. This is especially true when the reasons for it are hidden in the past or involve an emotional event that we think we have dealt with or that is long behind us. Our father saying to us, "You will never amount to anything," may have instilled a deep-seated fear that we are doomed to failure in anything we try. Look at your behavior and see if you've developed any rituals or patterns that consistently sabotage your progress. Do you consistently "forget" to meet with the boss? Do you consistently find yourself turning in a project or report after the deadline? At home, do you begin a project only to make some silly error that could have been avoided? Do you lose yourself in a novel rather than returning a call from your child's teacher? When these types of behaviors indicate a pattern, that is the time to look at the idea of self-sabotage. It might be helpful to put the way you self-sabotage in the middle of a piece of paper and then look at all the "whys" that radiate from it.

Tap into a mentor for insight and a reality check:

We can't always see the forest for the trees as to how or why we're self-sabotaging. There are times you'll need to trust a wiser head to point out the places and ways you're shooting yourself in the foot.

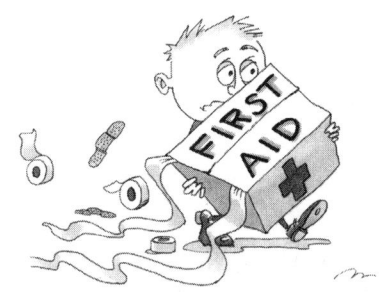

Need More First Aid?

Whether you are into self-sabotage or not, is the world just too much? If so, check out:

Chapter 1 on Overwhelm.

Do bills, taxes, credit cards

cause you problems? Part of your pattern of self-sabotage maybe solved by learning about:

Money in Chapter 12.

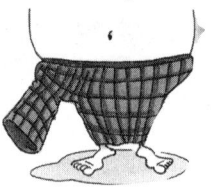

Do you feel so lost and blue that it's impossible to haul yourself out of bed in the morning? If so, look up:

Depression in Chapter 17.

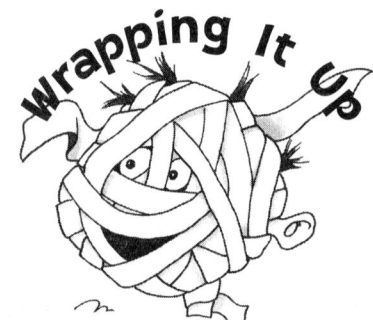

- Self-sabotage typically takes two forms: not taking action when action is needed, and holding onto negative thoughts and feelings.

- When we are in trouble, self-sabotage is usually the last thing we consider. After all, "Why would we do this to ourselves?"

- Self-sabotage can easily encompass elements of problems with money, difficulty in organizing, and depression.

- The first task is to identify the brick wall or stumbling block.

- Once self-sabotage is identified as the culprit, specific techniques will move you through the process.

> "Come out of the victim position and realize that you have the ability to put yourself in control of your actions and your thoughts. It's a conscious choice. Empower yourself!"
>
> *-Joan and Denise*

Late Again

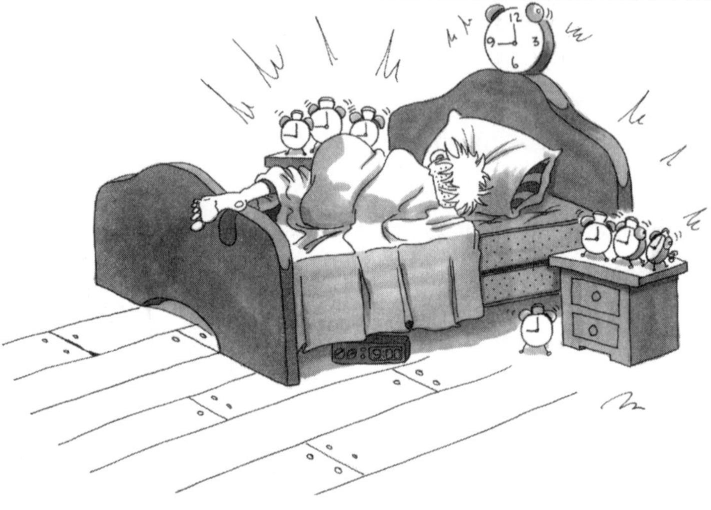

Chapter 14

What You Need To Know

Adults with SOP often have trouble with time. In fact, we may be operating in a world where a distorted sense of "AESOP time" rules rather than the "real time" used by the rest of the population. Scientific research suggests that our actual time sense may be distorted due to a dop-amine imbalance in our brains. No matter what the reason, this puts us out of sync with the rest of the world, and others misperceive our lateness as being inconsiderate, flaunting authority, or being downright rude.

Compounding the chemical impact on time are two pronounced AESOP traits. One is feeling an overwhelming urge to accomplish just one more task, water one more plant, make just one more phone call before we leave the house. We have no sense that each act takes time and will contribute to the lateness. In addition, the

> "Sooner or later, I'll be punctual."
> *-Ashleigh Brilliant*

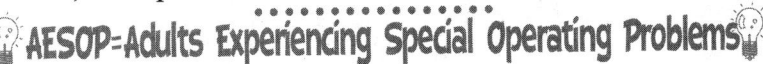

AESOP=Adults Experiencing Special Operating Problems

time it takes to do each additional task usually places us exactly the same number of minutes late to each subsequent event. Adults with SOP will invariably be exactly five minutes late, ten minutes late or fifteen minutes late. This leads the non-SOP world to think that if we can control the number of minutes we are late we can just as easily control our overall "lateness." In the AESOP world this is not true.

> *"The clock is always slow; it's later than you think."*
> —Robert Service

At times, Adults with SOP have developed a defensive attitude about their lateness. Do any of these sound familiar? "It's OK to be late because (pick one): I work late, I work through lunch, I don't take breaks." "My boss is going to be mad at me anyway, so why should I hurry into work?" "It won't matter if I'm late to the party, I'm not important anyway." "I already have a reputation for being late, why change it now?" If you know you have an attitude about your lateness, you'd best work on it because it will get in the way of your personal relationships and overall success in life.

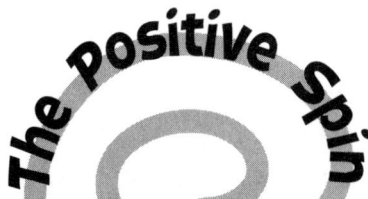
The Positive Spin

Realize that AESOPs may have a legitimate problem with time. Realize that being late or missing a deadline doesn't mean we're bad people or that we don't care. Know that by bringing our body chemistries into balance and using various techniques we can help ourselves work within realistic time frames.

Techniques
Getting Up

Practice mind control:

Shift your thoughts from "What time do I need to be there?" to "What time do I have to leave here?" Focus your mind on the clock with tunnel vision that says, "By this time, I need to be gone."

Plan ahead:

Set the coffee timer so coffee is made automatically. Stock easy-to-assemble breakfast foods. If you eat in the car, consider extra napkins (or a bib). The principle here is to grab and run. Get the things you'll need to take with you ready the night before and place them by the front door or in the car. DON'T PROMISE YOURSELF YOU'LL GET UP EARLY AND DO ANYTHING IN THE MORNING!

Collect tools for your toolbox:

Set up your crucial carry-all. Have a designated bag for all your needs on a day-to-day basis, (i.e., daytimer, pens, paper, cellular phone, timer, breath mints, money, I.D., etc.). Before you go to sleep, place this bag by the door, ready to pick up and go.

Investigate alarm clocks:

Notice we use the plural! Buy alarm clocks of varying pitch and intensity. We quickly become immune to the sound produced by only one alarm clock. Set alarm clocks around the room at increasing distances from your bed so you must get up. Consider alternatives to traditional alarms. There are alarm clocks that produce increasing amounts of light instead of sound to wake you up, as well as alarm clocks that vibrate you awake.

they go about their work of stabilizing the system, have a positive effect on sleep. For some AESOPs, a stimulant

> *"Decide to get up thirty minutes earlier. Do this for a year, and you will add seven and one-half days to your waking world."*
>
> -*Life's Little Treasure Book On Success*

Use medication to help you:

Adults with SOP frequently have had various medications prescribed to help their body chemistry re-balance itself. Many of these medications, as medication can be part of the treatment package. If this is true for you, set one alarm for half an hour before you need to get up. When the alarm goes off, take the medication you have placed on the night stand the night before. This lets the medication enter your system over the next half hour to help you wake up to the next alarm and be your best productive self.

Recognize the night owl syndrome:

If you are truly a night owl, accept your body's rhythm and realize you may need to search out a job where you can work on the swing or graveyard shift. Consider changing your job so that you don't have time constraints; for example, move to outside sales or something else without definite hours.

Analyze your bed time:

How many hours of sleep do you need each night to feel good or to be at your best? Be sure you get to bed in time to meet your sleep goal.

Attitude Adjustment

Be honest with yourself:

Do you have an attitude about your lateness? If so, where did your attitude or resentment start? Why did you become defensive? Did others' comments start to eat at your self-esteem? Did you give up trying to operate in "real time"?

Be honest with others:

Once you have identified an attitude about lateness and have decided to work on it, don't hesitate to let others know that it's been a problem you're trying to change. You may end up enlisting their help instead of their criticism.

Accept the real world:

Remember, AESOPs make up only a small percent of the population. You must survive in the "real world."

Be responsible for yourself:

The non-AESOP world doesn't understand what you go through on a daily basis in order to get to work, maintain a family, and exist in the world. Don't expect this understanding. Instead, take control of your own life. Be sure you provide time for

> "People who are late are often so much jollier than the people who have to wait for them."
> -E.V. Lucas

AESOP=Adults Experiencing Special Operating Problems

fun, relaxation, and spiritual growth.

 Appreciate your uniqueness:

As you are struggling just to get to work on time, remember to appreciate the creativity and uniqueness that encompasses the positive, "up" side to being an AESOP.

Don't hesitate to apologize:

If you have snapped at someone who commented on your lateness but didn't deserve to have their head bitten off, go back to them and apologize once you've cooled off.

Smile and the whole world smiles with you:

If you're out of sorts and grumpy, sometimes putting on a smile helps you make it through the day. It may actually improve your attitude and mental framework. Remember, it really does take more muscles to frown than it does to smile.

Chapter 14 • Late Again

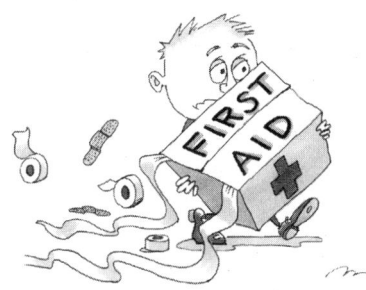

Need More First Aid?

If being late is caused by how you manage time, see:
Time Management in Chapter 5.

If you find that you just can't get out of the door, check out:

Chapter 6 on Procrastination.

If your particular brand of lateness is caused by your sleep pattern (or overall lack of sleep), see:
Chapter 31 on Sleep.

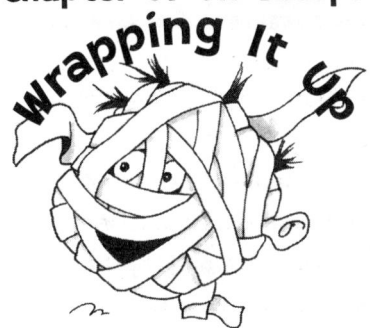

- Even Adults with SOP must realize that they live in

the real world and are bound by the constraints of "real time."

- Variations in body chemistry, depth of sleep, and even attitudes toward being late definitely affect this tendency to be "late again," and again, and again.

- Meet the challenge of being late head-on. Consider the role that body chemistry plays in your life, and use specific techniques that will make a definite difference.

Chapter 14 • Late Again

> "Know that by bringing our body chemistries into balance and using various techniques we can help ourselves work within realistic time frames."
> —*Joan and Denise*

Foot-In-Mouth Syndrome

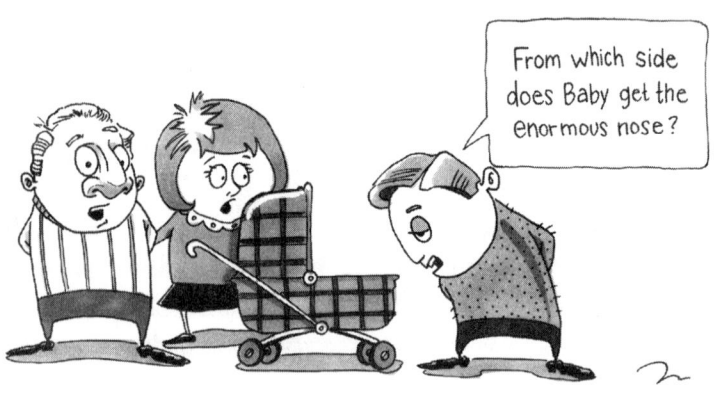

Chapter 15

What You Need To Know

The "Foot-in-Mouth" syndrome is experienced in two ways. The first is the sinking sensation in the pit of your stomach when you've just said something and you hear how it came out. You find yourself thinking, "I can't believe I just said that. What is wrong with me?" The second is the sinking sensation you have in the pit of your stomach when you see someone's expression, and you know you have made a horrible blunder. You think, "What did I say? Why are they upset?" or more often, "I can't remember what I just said." Too often impulsivity and trouble with social cues are the root causes of "Foot-in-Mouth" syndrome.

The Positive Spin

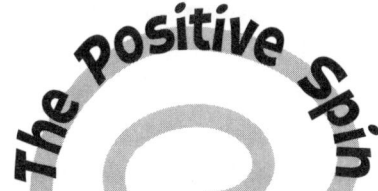

Down deep inside you know you are a good person. Your inner motives are pure. You wouldn't hurt anyone for the world. Remind yourself that

AESOP=Adults Experiencing Special Operating Problems

having your foot in your mouth is an awkward position, not a moral flaw. It is a problem that can be identified, modified, and resolved.

Techniques

Pre-plan and practice:

For important conversations, decide what you want to say in advance. Next, choose the best method of delivery: phone, face to face, email, or letter. Make notes, then write a script that makes your point. Practice your script in front of a mirror. Consider recording it so you can hear yourself. Remember, rehearsal leads to a better performance.

Get a grip on yourself:

Create a space for yourself of three to five seconds prior to launching into a conversation. This gives you time to center yourself, and to assess whether you're going to come across the way that you want. This space can be created by deep breathing or by something as simple as crossing your fingers to remind yourself to slow down. This technique can be especially useful when you feel angry, or when you feel your blood pressure or stress level rising.

Bone up on social cues:

Reading social cues is a skill you can learn. Take a class at the local college; buy a book or a tape on the subject.

> "I always know the right thing to say, after the right time to say it has passed."
> -Ashleigh Brilliant

Select a mentor who will teach you about social cues without shaming you. Lastly, observe, observe, observe. The great anthropologist Margaret Mead learned about tribes by quietly observing them and recording their behavior before joining in. In this way she could be sure that she wasn't making social blunders that would offend anyone in the tribe. Think of non-AESOPs as an alien and unknown tribe. Watch closely, then leap in for the best chance to blend.

Learn re-opening:

When you have had a conversation that didn't go as planned, it is perfectly accept-

> "The passion for setting people right is in itself an afflictive disease."
> -Marianne Moore

able to approach the person you spoke with and ask whether the conversation can be re-opened. Consider saying: "Yesterday when we talked, I didn't express myself the way that I wanted. I'd like to re-visit the conversation," or "You know the conversation we had earlier? What I wanted to say was..." If your AESOP status is known and accepted, try, "Yesterday was one of my AESOP days. I hope what I said didn't offend you. I'd like to talk about that particular topic again."

Practice the graceful exit:

When you have dug yourself in so deep that no immediate redemption is possible, sometimes the only solution is to exit gracefully. At times you may need only three or four minutes alone in order to collect yourself. Phrases such as "Would you excuse me for a moment, I need to make a phone call," or "I need to use the restroom" can do the trick. For those "Oh my God, what have I done?" situations, use a phrase such as "I just noticed the time and have to hurry to get to an appointment." Alternatively, look startled, then look down at your pager as though the vibration has signaled you. This enables you to make a quick exit.

The day after:

If you have had to use "The Graceful Exit" technique, you may be painfully aware that you have caused hurt feelings. You may fear that you have irreparably damaged a friendship, or you may feel so rotten about what you have said that you can't live with yourself. The temptation to stick your head in the sand and ignore the incident will be strong. But in the long run, this is a mistake; your feelings won't

> "If A equals success, then the formula is A=X+Y+Z. X is work. Y is play. Z is keep your mouth shut."
>
> *-Albert Einstein*

> **"Remember that how you say something is as important as what you say."**
>
> -*Life's Little Treasure Book On Wisdom*

go away, they will remain and nag at you over time. If too much time elapses before you make any attempt at communication, it becomes much more difficult to correct the situation.

No matter how much you wish the incident would go away, it won't. This is time to take action. Try a phone call; open the conversation with, "I've been thinking about what I said to you yesterday and I'm afraid that I hurt your feelings." Or try this: "Driving home, I realized that I came off totally wrong. I really care about you, and I wouldn't have hurt you for the world. Let me try and explain what I meant."

If the thought of approaching the phone is beyond you, resort to a note. Write it; then (this is important!) let it sit on

Chapter 15 • Foot-In-Mouth Syndrome

your desk for twenty-four hours before actually slipping it in the mail. This allows you time to think about what you have said and re-write if necessary. If writing your feelings on paper is impossible for you, there still is a solution at hand. Your local bookstore will carry a book or two full of sample letters to be used for all sorts of occasions. Select a letter dealing with an apology or message of sympathy with words or phrases that come close to what you feel in your heart and that you desperately wish you could express. Add a phrase or change a word or two and the job is done.

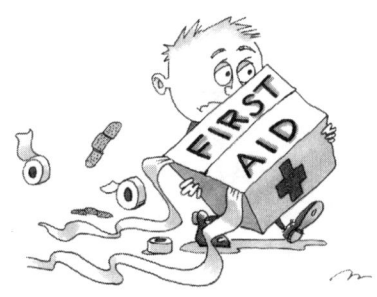

Need More First Aid?

If the pressures of work or obligations at home have you running 100 miles an hour,

you may need to slow down, see:
Chapter 5 on Time Management.

If you tend to jump in no matter what, see:
Impulsivity, in Chapter 9.

If part of your problem centers around your habit of floating off and then jumping in (with your foot in your mouth), check out:
Chapter 10 on Distractibility.

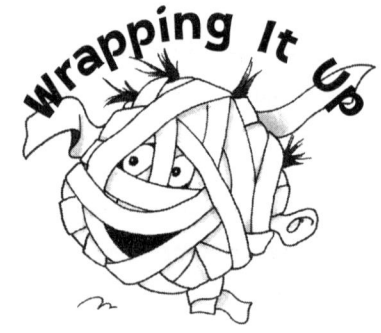

Wrapping It Up

- The Foot-in-Mouth Syndrome can be experienced in two ways: you may know immediately you have made a blunder or you may see the horrified expressions around you and *then* realize that you have made a blunder.

- Affirm to yourself that you

are a good and kind person (or you wouldn't care enough to be reading this chapter).

- Identify what is contributing to your habit of finding your foot in your mouth and take steps to remove it.

- At times, even with the best of plans you will still find your foot in your mouth. At those times, use a technique such as "the graceful exit" to extricate yourself.

- Do your best to lighten it up and keep a little humor in any situation. After all, who else uses the "startled pager trick" to make a graceful exit?

- Remind yourself YOU ARE A GOOD PERSON! Remember to tell yourself that the pattern does not constitute a moral flaw and ask others for this same understanding.

> "Having your foot in your mouth is an awkward position, not a moral flaw."
> *-Joan and Denise*

Moods

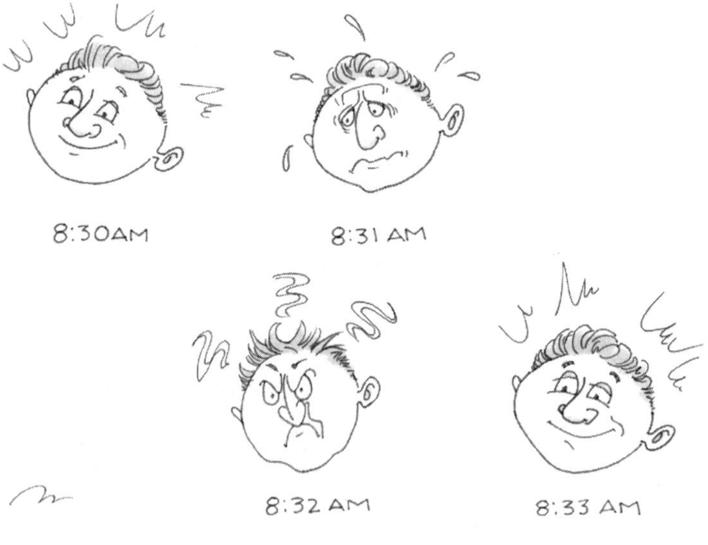

8:30 AM

8:31 AM

8:32 AM

8:33 AM

Chapter 16

What You Need To Know

Human beings are creatures of mood. Whether linked with the moon, the tides, our menstrual cycles, or the time of year, moods are part and parcel of our make-up. Over the years the Adult with SOP may have gotten a reputation for being moody, excitable, extreme, or quick to go from highs to lows. The trouble occurs when moods either become excessive or hang around for too long. At the opposite end of the spectrum, some AESOPs may experience a total absence of mood or emotion, appearing flat and lifeless, which is a problem in itself.

The Positive Spin

While excessive moods can cause trouble, let's take a look at the "up" side. It's this quicksilver spirit that often gives Adults with SOP their creativity, flashes of brilliance and zest for life. A positive approach is to celebrate that quicksilver

AESOP=Adults Experiencing Special Operating Problems

spirit while learning how to balance and temper our moods.

Techniques

Adjusting Body Chemistry

Exercise can be key:

If we have a tendency toward super-high or super-low energy, exercise can help normalize both ends of the spectrum. Aerobic exercise actually alters the brain chemistry by activating the endorphin system. To have this endorphin-enhancing effect, the exercise must be both rigorous and aerobic; it must engage the cardio-vascular system, increasing heart rate and respiration. A good example is running three miles consistently. Weight training, while certainly good for you, will not have the same mood-altering effect.

Herbs or vitamins:

If we wake up really feeling blue and end the day really "up" or vice versa, our body may be deficient in certain minerals or vitamins. A good multi-vitamin with certain supplements added may improve your overall health.

> "I say if it's going to be done, let's do it. Let's not put it in the hands of fate. Let's not put it in the hands of someone who doesn't know me. I know me best. Then take a breath and go ahead."
>
> *-Anita Baker*

This in turn may help to stabilize moods. Certain herbs, such as St. John's Wort, are promoted as natural remedies for moods. If this approach seems to be the right one for you, develop a relationship with the owner of your local health food store. If even more expertise is needed, consult a specialist in herbal medicine. However, be aware that there are an overwhelming number of homeopathic "remedies" on the shelves of your local health food store. Sometimes it's better to start with a reasonable program outlined in a book written by a person who seems to have the expertise required (check the author's bio for their education and level of expertise). Often our friendly health food store owner or a particularly astute friend can point us in the right direction.

Consider Eastern medicine:

If vitamins and minerals or herbs alone are not quite doing the job, consider visiting an acupuncturist with the expertise to soften mood changes or to control mood balance. Experts in Eastern medicine will not only use acupuncture but also have a sophisticated knowledge of herbs at their disposal.

Consider Western medicine:

Sometimes if our chemistry is far enough out of whack,

> "The limbic emotional system is intimately tied in with the immune system, and being able to develop and express our emotions allows us a healthy life."
> -Carla Hannaford

Chapter 16 • Moods

Western medication may be the fastest and most effective way to regulate moods. Remember the use of medication to treat brain chemistry imbalances is no more a sign of failure than is using medication to treat obvious physical ailments such as allergies or headaches. It is a positive step to recognize that our body chemistry may benefit from this type of support.

Further Mood Regulators

Be aware of your diet and food allergies:

Some AESOPs have obvious responses to certain foods that plunge them into mood swings. Signs to look for are dramatic responses to foods. For example, if sugar makes you extremely hyperactive, extremely sleepy, or makes you crave more and more sugar, this is a sure sign that there is something going on. If a large plate of pasta makes you head right toward the couch for a nap or, more telling, sets you obsessing about the pan of Rice Krispies treats on the counter (made for the Girl Scout meeting tomorrow), you may be having an allergic response. The danger here is beginning a cycle. If you are allergic to a certain substance, one portion may trigger a whole series of cravings, leaving you with even more to battle. The rule? Stay away from foods that cause you problems. Remember, we're often drawn to foods that we are allergic to. If you're not sure whether any of these patterns fit you, ask your partner, family, or friends. Finally, if you're still not sure, get allergy tested.

> "Pay as much attention to the things that are working positively in your life as you do to those that are giving you trouble."
> —*Life's Little Treasure Book On Wisdom*

Chapter 16 • Moods

Pay attention to your sleep:

Get to know what your body needs. Both too much and too little sleep can contribute to mood problems. If your sleep problems are severe, consider that you may have sleep apnea or another medical problem that disrupts sleep, and get a medical opinion from a specialist.

Develop your use of meditation or prayer:

Humans have always turned to a Higher Power to link themselves with feelings of safety, to feel grounded, to make sense of things that seem senseless. For some people, this means being involved with a particular religion or belief. For others, meditation comes from sitting quietly or walking on the beach or in a forest. The setting and structure can be formal or informal; just do it.

At times, the formal ritual of a yoga class or a meditation group that meets at a certain time each week helps to establish a routine in your life that will allow you to continue whichever method you choose.

Use water to help balance:

We are made up of water and benefit from taking it into our bodies or being around or in it. Diving into a pool, taking a bubble bath, or drinking a tall glass of water all help.

Consider cognitive therapy:

Moods occur primarily in the limbic system, the emotion center of the brain. Cognitive therapy using active problem-solving techniques forces us to move out of our emotions and into our logic center to deal with our emotions on a cognitive level. There are self-help books on cognitive therapy in the bookstore or library. There are also psychologists who specialize in this type of therapy; for starters, try the yellow pages.

Use support groups:

When you're feeling terrible, nothing helps like talking to someone who's had the same experiences and can connect with you on the basic level of "Yes, I've been there." Don't be afraid to sample more than one group before you find the right people for you. It's worth it! Sometimes support groups for "moods" or "depression" are not easy to locate. Remember that any group, whether it is a local book discussion group or a group of gardeners, offers the strong possibility that you will run into a soul mate. Be aware that developing this type of connection with another person may take time. They may be hesitant to share or open up, especially if they are in pain (as you are). Have patience with the process.

> "I don't wait for moods. You accomplish nothing if you do that. Your mind must know it has got to get down to earth."
> -*Pearl S. Buck*

Use music:

Music can transport us to a different awareness or emotion. It can help replace sadness with joy; the pulse of a beat or the softness of the sounds can elevate or soothe. For some, music is the equivalent of meditation.

Tune into yourself:

Be aware of what different environments do to you. If visual stimuli or busy, noisy places drive you crazy, consider avoiding county fairs, malls, shopping centers, and places that would set you off. Think of alternatives such as shopping by catalogue, attending a quieter concert, or choosing events with fewer people attending. Take care of yourself.

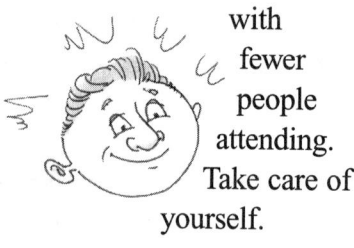

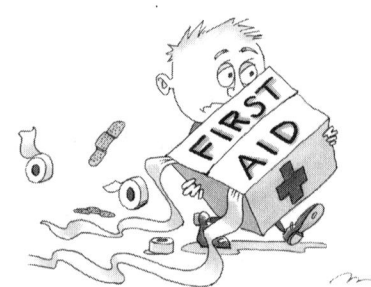

Need More First Aid?

If your moods seem to be triggered by stress in your life, see:

Chapter 2 on Stress Reduction and Chapter 28 on Balance in Life.

Chapter 16 • Moods

If your moods erupt into angry outbursts, see:
Chapter 19 on Anger.

If grief and loss are significant contributors to your moods, see:
Chapter 20 on Grief.

If you are still having problems with moods and aren't sure if there's something else going on, see:
Chapter 35 on Co-Occurring Conditions.

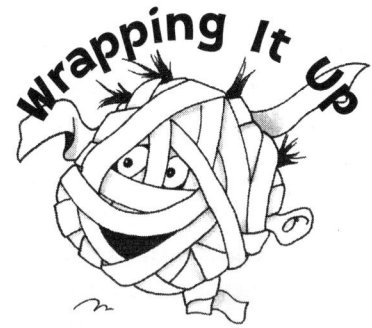

- Moods are definitely part of the human condition.

- It is only when they become excessive or out of control that they upset our emotional health and our productivity.

- The object is not to eliminate moods, but to moderate

or soften them.

- A variety of techniques including exercise, herbal remedies Eastern or Western medicine, and cognitive therapy offers a range of effective possibilities for treatment.

- Take a good look at yourself. Decide which treatment approach to pursue. If the first approach doesn't work, pick another approach or a combination of several approaches and try again.

Chapter 16 • Moods

> "While excessive moods can cause trouble, let's take a look at the "up" side. It's this quicksilver spirit that often gives Adults with SOP their creativity, flashes of brilliance and zest for life."
>
> —*Joan and Denise*

Depression

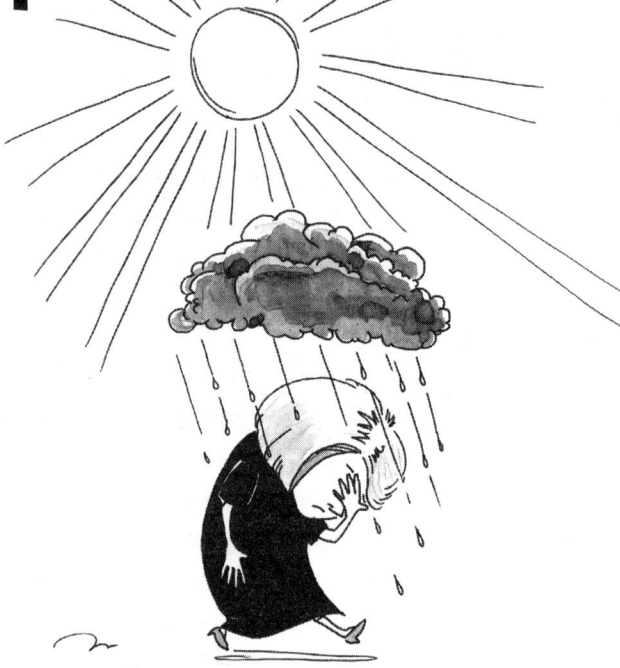

Chapter 17

What You Need To Know

The world seems flat and gray. Nothing entices you to move off the couch; in fact, a nap seems the best idea going. You feel you have no motivation. Could it be depression? This word may seem too severe for what you are feeling, but depression is what it may be.

Many AESOPs suffer from a long-standing, low-grade depression without ever putting a name to it. This depression can have at least two possible origins. One is that the depression is chemically caused by a lack of serotonin in the brain. This type of depression often begins in childhood and is never named or diagnosed; as an adult you may view this state of mind as simply "normal." The second possible cause of depression for AESOPs can be the remembrance of past hurts or failures in school or in life. This can include a sense of hopelessness, a feeling that you have never reached your potential in relationships or career, and a fear

AESOP=Adults Experiencing Special Operating Problems

that you probably never will.

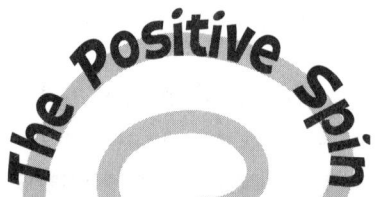

The Positive Spin

Once depression is identified and named, then you can begin to find solutions. You are no longer fighting a shapeless gray cloud that brings your life to a halt. Is your depression chemical or is it caused by thinking about past events? Is it a little of both? Be aware there is often an overlapping of these two causes, and both must be identified. Once you have identified the possible causes of your depression, you will be able to move in the right direction to make positive changes.

Techniques
Biochemical Depression

Check out the level of depression:

If you sense your level of depression is escalating, don't wait for it to get worse to bring it to your physician's attention. If you feel incapacitated by your depression, arrange to see your family doctor or psychiatrist immediately to discuss the advisability of medication. There are many new types of antidepressants now available with minimal side effects.

Start cardiovascular exercise:

Running, biking, or walking will change body chemistry and help to lift depression. It doesn't take long for the change to be apparent; often within a week or two, the depression seems to be lighter. For AESOPs, the trick is to maintain the exercise. Remember, having an exercise buddy or a support system helps.

Consider herbal remedies:

These seem to appear and disappear from the shelves of your local health food store with bewildering frequency. At times they provide some relief. However, you need to be aware that herbs can actually be more dangerous than prescription drugs. For one thing, there is little quality control over their manufacturing. People often think that because herbs are natural substances they are somehow a

> "Life is often hard. You can let it grind you down or polish you up."
>
> -Life's Little Treasure Book On Hope

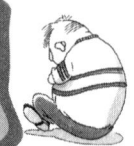

safer choice, and may even go on the premise that "more is better." Consider looking for a professional such as a holistic physician or acupuncturist with herbal experience. Also, if you choose to experiment with herbal remedies let your prescribing physician and/or pharmacist know so they can check for incompatibilities or drug interactions.

Do you need vitamins?

These, taken in a balanced formula, increase general health. If you are healthy, your whole body--including your brain--functions in better balance, and depression may be alleviated. Be careful of megadoses of vitamins as well.

Consider Eastern medicine:

The East has amassed centuries of knowledge in the art of healing. Depression can often be improved with the help of

Chapter 17 • Depression

licensed acupuncturists or other Eastern medicine practitioners who typically prescribe a blend of herbs specifically formulated for each individual.

Use other professionals:

Chiropractors and massage therapists are often very helpful in alleviating depression. Practitioners in both of these areas have expertise far beyond relaxing sore or aching muscles. Their treatment includes techniques that balance or adjust energy fields. If energy fields are aligned correctly, it is as though channels are unblocked, which then allows the body to heal itself. Depression often causes the body to have a sluggish or heavy feeling. Treatment facilitates the moving of this negative field or energy.

Consider other alternatives:

Meditation and yoga, practiced regularly, change brain waves and can also lift depression.

Depression from Life Events

Identify possible origins of your depression:

Do memories of failures in

school haunt you? Did you have trouble getting along with classmates? Did teachers misunderstand your type of special operating problems and make critical or hurtful comments? Were you told that you would never make it in college by your high school counselor? Did these past situations leave scars? Remember, sadness turned inward can cause depression. Or is the depression centered more on your current situation? Are there problems at work or in your relationships? All of these life events can cause depression.

Join a 12-Step Program:

12-Step groups can be found for almost any problem that you can think of. Don't be afraid to try them out. These groups follow a 12-step stan-

> "When you are worried, give your troubles to God or a higher power. He will be up all night anyway."
> -Life's Little Treasure Book On Hope

dard format and are helpful when working through specific hurts.

Meet other AESOPs:

12-Step groups as well as conferences regarding your specific SOP provide a forum for meeting other adults who have experienced many of the same problems. As you run into people in these settings, you'll often find one or two with whom you feel a real kinship. These are the ones you'll want to spend time with. Often nothing helps as much as someone else saying, "I know how you feel. I've been through it too."

Learn about your own Special Operating Problems:

This sounds like a trite solution, but it is actually vital. Check the bookstores, the Internet, the library, the Calendar section of your newspaper for information. When you understand the full scope of your SOP, both the positives and the negatives, it allows you to understand yourself. You can then treat yourself with greater kindness and forgiveness. This gives you the freedom to expand your horizons and look for new and creative ways to alleviate depression.

Broaden your information base to the national level:

Try one of the national conferences where a number of presenters gather to provide two or three days chock full of information. Join a local or national organization related to your SOP and be alert for upcoming events. To find information on conferences, check the Internet. Sign up for newsletters that deal with your specific type of SOP. Advertisements about conferences will often appear in these publications and no where else.

Handle past hurts:

If you can't get that awful teacher you had as a freshman in high school out of your mind, try journal writing to relieve the pain. Buy a notebook or journal. Promise yourself time each day to actually write. (Setting aside the same time each day, either first thing in the morning or just before bedtime helps establish it as a habit.) Be sure to secure the journal in a safe place where whatever you write remains yours alone. No matter how long ago the event occurred, write a letter to your teacher telling him or her how much their actions or comments hurt you. The purpose of the letter is to release these emotions that you are carrying around. The success of this technique is not dependent on a reply.

However, at times this is a bonus, as a teacher (who was well meaning, but dead wrong about your abilities) will write you a sincere letter of apology.

The last technique involves writing a letter that you may choose not to send or may not be able to send if the offend-

> "Worry makes for a hard pillow. When something's troubling you, before going to sleep, jot down three things you can do the next day to solve the problem."
> -*Life's Little Treasure Book On Wisdom*

ing party has passed away. This helps to distance you from the pain. Once the letter is written, if it is not mailed, send it to the person symbolically. Burn the letter and scatter the ashes from a cliff. Tear the letter into pieces and flush it down the toilet. It isn't important that it be received by the person, but that you've released it into the universe.

Remember past hurts:

Another possibility: Write a letter, as an adult, to yourself when you were a child or teenager. Target the time period that evokes the most emotion as you think about your life. Write kindly to yourself, offering sympathy and reassurance as well as a hope for the future. This often acts as though a sympathetic friend has put an arm around you and said, "I understand you had a tough time." A sample of such a letter might be from Sarah the adult to Sarah the child

Chapter 17 • Depression

and might begin like this:

> Dear Sarah,
>
> As I look back from my wisdom of forty five years of life and look at you as a ten year old I have tears running down my cheeks. You were so sad and lonely. So many nights were spent crying yourself to sleep because no one could understand you. I know you didn't see your moods and depression for what they were. Instead they made up one big ball of hurt. I know the times you said mean things to your sister weren't really because you hated her (like you said), but it seemed like she had everything (good grades, boy friends, long straight hair) and you had nothing.

Deal with hurts you have done to others:

In their pain and anger, children with special operating problems may often have hit a classmate or said mean things. As an adult, this often sits on your shoulders as a load of heavy guilt. There are several ways to make amends. One involves recognizing that much of your behavior may have been beyond your control and deciding to simply stop being so hard on yourself. Another method involves writing a letter or contacting that person with an apology. (This is actually one of the 12 Steps, "Making Amends," but it can certainly be done separately.) If neither of these actions seems appropriate, sometimes giving back to the universe by being a Big Brother or Big Sister or working with an organization such as Habitat for Humanity can make you feel that you are balancing the scales of life.

Tackle hopelessness about the future:

You still can't see a clear path ahead for yourself. Instead, because the path is confusing, you have a tendency to pull back, shut down, and let depression take over. This facet of depression must be met with a proactive attitude. Break the roadblocks down into smaller components, attack each one in isolation, and set small goals for yourself. Get moving!

> **"Despair doubles our strength."**
> *-French Proverb*

Have a coach:

A close friend, family member, or a loved one can help you clearly evaluate or define your feelings. When we are in pain we often can't achieve the perspective we need. Asking someone we trust, "Am I off base? Am I too angry?" can help us see more clearly. They can also help us channel our feelings by simply listening or offering another way of looking at life.

Consider counseling or professional help:

Professionals often assist you in relieving depression more quickly; they can speed up the process of identifying the difficulty and moving toward a solution. Often we delay this step as we try all other options; however, this shouldn't be considered as a last resort. Counseling with someone who specializes in AESOPs is money well-spent.

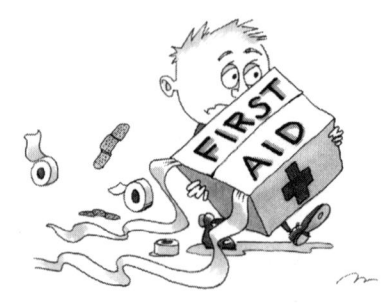

Need More First Aid?

If guilt is pervasive in your life and sits on you like a heavy stone, see:
Shame and Guilt in Chapter 18.

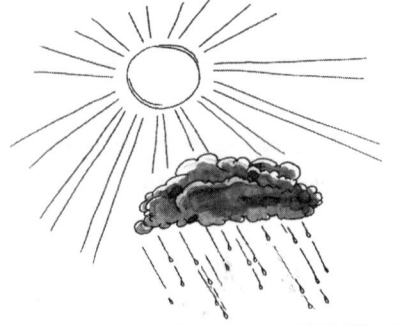

If depression is not the only feeling you struggle with, see:
Moods in Chapter 16.

If starting or maintaining an exercise program is difficult for you, see:
Exercise in Chapter 30.

If you recognize that you are depressed, but sense that something else is also interfering with your life, see:
Co-Occurring Conditions in Chapter 35.

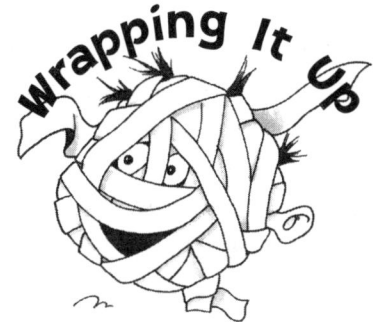

Wrapping It Up

- Depression can be caused by a biochemical imbalance in your system.

- Depression can also come from current glitches in your life or the burden of carrying around unresolved past hurts.

- Depression *can* be a combination of the two, and in fact is *very often* a combination of the two.

● Once the cause for depression is identified, the strategies for dealing with it become more clear.

● Treatment by your physician or psychiatrist may be a vital part of alleviating depression.

● Depression happens to all of us at certain points in our lives. It is part of the human condition and can become dangerous or incapacitating when it is ignored. Tackle it head-on.

> "Once depression is identified and named, then you can begin to find solutions. You are no longer fighting a shapeless gray cloud that brings your life to a halt."
>
> *-Joan and Denise*

Shame and Guilt

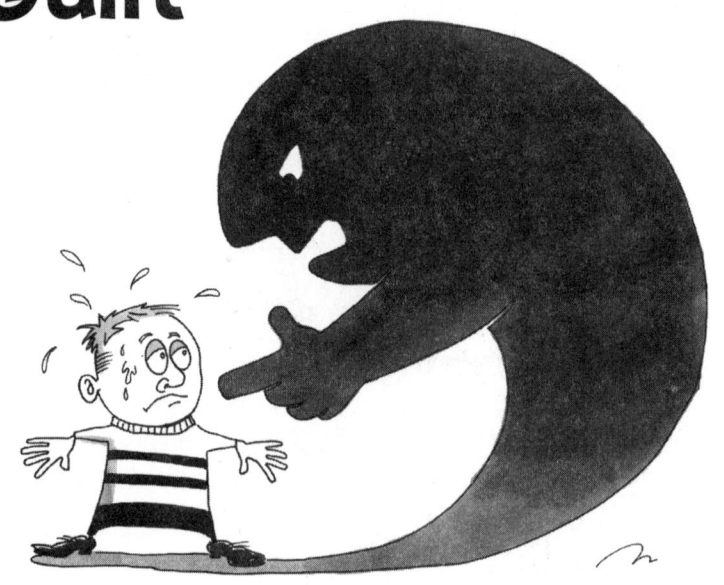

Chapter 18

What You Need To Know

Guilt is a feeling that results from having done something you feel is wrong. Shame is the feeling inside yourself, that says you are flawed as a person, not worthy, really bad to the bone. When AESOPs look back on things they haven't done or people they've hurt, they often feel that they're simply not good enough or smart enough; they just can't reach the mark. Because guilt and shame may be pervasive feelings among AESOPs, we need to understand that many of the actions or perceptions that cause our shame and guilt can be chalked up to chemistry that is out of balance.

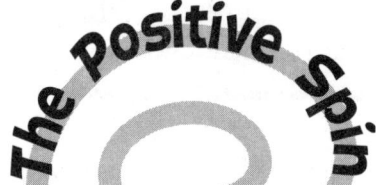

Shame: Who we are is made up of how we grew up, where we grew up, who was around us, what we were taught, and our body chemistries. Often the body chemistry of an AESOP is what tilts the scale and

AESOP=Adults Experiencing Special Operating Problems

throws the other stuff out of balance.

Guilt: What we do is related to the choices we make. These choices are strongly influenced by all of the above factors. Resolving guilt is an action phase; we must do something to correct our previous actions or inaction.

Shame and guilt are very personal feelings. We can work successfully with these feelings to bring ourselves a sense of peace. This peace includes that deep internal sigh of relief, the sense that all the demons have been put to rest.

Techniques
Handling Shame

Practice separating Self from Behavior:

"Who I am" versus "what I do" are the questions at issue. We often confuse these two very separate ideas without taking the time to see how destructive this is to our sense of ourselves and to our self-esteem. Here is an exercise to help you practice this separation: Take a piece of paper and create two columns, one marked "Who I am" and one "What I do." Choose a situation that you haven't been comfortable with and consider carefully whether the discomfort you feel is about what you've done or not done (which can often be corrected) versus who you are (which requires deeper examination).

Establish or reestablish a connection with God or your Higher Power:

This affirms your innate goodness. God the Creator didn't create you as a lesser person; and it's important to realize that experiencing special operating problems in your life does not in any way diminish your true goodness.

Make a list of positive traits:

If our feelings of shame and guilt cause us to have problems doing this, we can ask trusted friends or family for input. Another avenue for discovering and listing positive traits is to note what we are not and work backward from there. An example might be "I'm not

> "Compassion for self is the most powerful healer of them all."
> -Theodore Isaac Rubin

a liar" which can be reexamined and reworded to "I am an honest person."

> "Mistakes are part of the dues one pays for a full life."
> -Sophia Loren

Use daily affirmations:

We can build in a daily routine of affirming our spiritual connections and ourselves. Consider putting positive traits on index cards and stating them in the present tense. Use strong, affirming language such as "I am a kind and loving person." "I am blessed by God (or my Higher Power) from within." Practicing these several times a day begins to reprogram a negative self-concept. Be persistent!

Take advantage of nature:

Go out into nature, to the mountains or the beach, and observe its perfection. Realize that we are an integral part of this beautiful creation. As each natural thing is made unique and complete in its own way, so, too, are we.

Reality check:

Locate a trusted person, a

friend, mentor or therapist, who can provide a reality check about our inner being. When our internal validation system doesn't feel like it's kicking in, a trusted outside source can help us get our positive self-thoughts started.

Share feelings of shame with other safe people:

Sharing our deepest pain and shame with other Adults with SOP often helps us normalize the feelings and put them into perspective. There can be tremendous relief in knowing we are not the only ones who may be walking around feeling ashamed of our inner feelings.

Handling Guilt

Practice separating your behavior from who you are:

Because of circumstances in our lives, which certainly can include problems with our body chemistry, we may truly have said or done things that have been harmful to others. If this is the case, it is important to take a compassionate look at ourselves as well as those we've hurt. Our inner worth cannot hinge solely upon our past deeds. However, a final step of making amends to repair things we've done or said can be important for healing.

Handling ghosts from the past:

Often we're plagued by events that happened in childhood or by interactions with people who have long been out of our lives. People automatically assume that there can be no resolution for these past events, yet even ancient history can be resolved and put to rest. People who are long gone, events that are well past can still be dealt with. Sometimes we can write a letter taking responsibility for a past action that was thoughtless or painful. Sometimes a phone call, a meeting, or even a quick note can begin to smooth the rough edges of something we've done and still feel badly about.

Identify your sources of guilt:

When guilt is a shadowy and pervasive feeling, we can't

do much about it. To get past that general feeling, try making a list of some things you feel guilty about right now, and select one thing at a time on which to start taking action and making head-way.

Ask yourself "What can I do about this?":

If something obvious comes to mind, decide whether to write a letter, make an appointment, or get on the phone to resolve this issue. Rehearse what you'll say before you make contact so you are well prepared to resolve rather than re-irritate.

As an example, you've missed an important meeting where your input was vital. Your tendency might be to act defensively. Rehearsing can modify that response to something like, "I am so sorry I missed our meeting earlier today. Can I put my feedback in writing and fax it over to

> "We have to learn to be our own best friends because we fall too easily into the trap of being our own worst enemies." -Roderick Thorp

you so can we still meet our deadline? I had really intended to be there and apologize if I caused any inconvenience."

If the situation can't be dealt with directly, ask yourself "What can I do to make amends?" If you can't go directly to the person or people involved, consider making amends through actions. Volunteer at an animal shelter, do community service, make a point of regularly saying something kind to someone who looks sad or worried.

If the person involved has died or moved away, we can still write them a letter. This allows us to release our feelings out to the universe. It provides us a place to take responsibility and ask for forgiveness. We need to take our time in writing this kind of letter. Imagine that this is the last chance we'll have to let this person know our perceptions, thoughts, and

> "A lie is an abomination unto the Lord and a very present help in time of trouble."
> -Adlai Stevenson

feelings. We must take responsibility for our actions where it's due. We must be as comprehensive as we can to provide as thorough a cleansing experience as possible. Sometimes burning the letter and scattering the ashes, or tearing the letter into tiny pieces and flushing them can provide further cleansing.

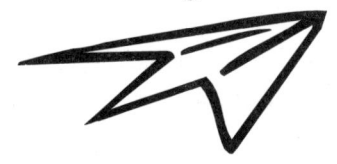

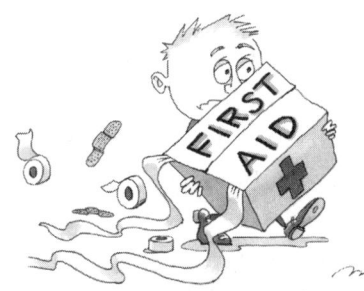

Need More First Aid?

If you have trouble with guilt because you're always doing or saying things that seem thoughtless or mean to others, see:
Foot-in-Mouth Syndrome in Chapter 15.

If shame and guilt have beaten you down, see:
Depression in Chapter 17.

If your actions have caused pain to you or people you care about, see:
Grief in Chapter 20.

If you have difficulty understanding or connecting with God or a Higher Power, see:
Spirituality in Chapter 34.

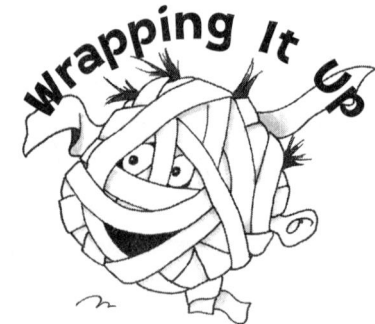

Wrapping It Up

- Feelings of guilt result from things we do or say; feelings of shame come from who we feel we are.

- Many Adults with SOP confuse and combine shame and guilt, resulting in a very poor concept of self.

- There are specific actions we can take to resolve guilt, whether the person is still in our lives or not.

- There are specific activities we can do to reinforce our sense of self and reduce our feelings of shame.

- Being able to separate guilt from shame and addressing each of them appropriately allows us to increase our sense of relief and peace.

> "Shame and guilt are very personal feelings. We can work successfully with these feelings to bring ourselves a sense of peace. This peace includes that deep internal sigh of relief, the sense that all the demons have been put to rest."
> *-Joan and Denise*

Anger

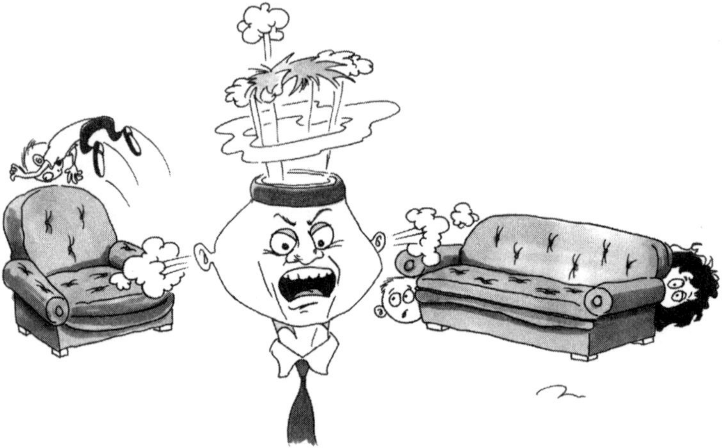

Chapter 19

What You Need To Know

In all of our lives there are things that cause us to feel angry: a fight with our spouse, a traffic jam, co-workers who don't pull their weight, always finding the slowest line in the supermarket. For the Adult with SOP, these common occurrences may cause even more distress because we are often struggling with a sense of low self-esteem, struggling to control rage, or struggling even to survive and balance our lives.

There is another component, which is anger caused by a bio-chemical imbalance. The levels of anger can range from a prickliness where everything irritates you to a wild swing of emotion that explodes into white-hot rage (inevitably followed by feelings of remorse or sadness).

Remember that there are two avenues for approaching the anger issue: one is through bio-chemical corrections, and the other is addressing the triggers that cause the anger.

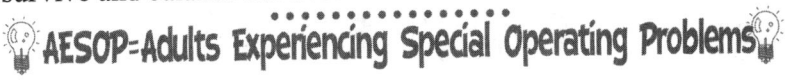
AESOP=Adults Experiencing Special Operating Problems

The Positive Spin

Be kind to yourself. Be aware that the anger you're dealing with is as much a part of your SOP as any other difficulty you might be experiencing, such as depression. As you work with your anger in this way, allow yourself to eliminate the feelings of shame and guilt often associated with it. Learn to problem-solve anger provoking events. Deal with anger as a common AESOP trait. There is an old saying that anger in the right amount, at the right time, in the right place, directed at the right person "is a normal healthy emotion." It's the anger that spills out the sides that is unhealthy and needs to be worked with like any of our traits that run amuck. There are specific triggers to anger which you can get to know and master. It can be done!

Techniques
Self-Monitoring Tools

Be aware of sure-fire triggers:

If you don't get enough rest, if you don't keep food fuel in your human tank, if you are taking medication that helps with anger and you forget to take it, you may be setting yourself up for an anger outburst or rage attack.

Use HALT! (+H):

Try the following memory trick to help monitor how likely you are to get angry. Trouble lies ahead if these basic stressors are neglected. (And note: we added a second "H" which stands for HOT!)

Ask yourself: Are you Hungry, Angry, Lonely, Tired (or Hot)?

The message here is to HALT, and ask yourself if you've taken care of these basic needs. If not, get to it!

Consider sleep, food, meds, exercise:

As an alternative to HALT, we've broken down problem areas to self-monitor another way: Sleep, Food, Meds, Exercise.

Sleep: Deprivation or loss of sleep causes major problems. Guard your rest!

Food: Lack of consistent food intake or generally having a terrible diet weakens your entire system. Eat well.

Medication: A system out of balance is impossible to regulate. Consider medication or herbal remedies; do something to support your biochemistry!

Exercise: Are you exercising? A sluggish system prevents your chemistry from working properly. It's a scientific fact that exercising increases endorphins in the brain, which increase feelings of well-being. We have known several cases of injured athletes who experienced surges of anger that were not present when they could exercise.

Monitor your thoughts:

Begin to look at the thoughts that immediately precede the anger-producing event or action. Identify automatic thoughts that may cue anger from your past conditioning such as "That idiot's driving like a maniac. I ought to catch up and give him a piece of my mind."

Watch your effect on others:

Realize the effect your angry outbursts have on colleagues, friends, and loved ones. Remember that you can have some control over your anger. Instead of letting their responses and facial expressions cue you to more anger, use them to self-monitor.

> "Hitting the ceiling is the worst way to get up in the world."
> -*20,000 Quips and Quotes*

Often, seeing the cause-and-effect of your anger, as it leads to others' distress will serve as a powerful motivation to change.

When you're too angry:

Warn others around you as soon as you become aware that you're getting angry. Sometimes you'll only be able to give a five-second warning, but giving fair warning is part of taking control of your anger.

AESOP=Adults Experiencing Special Operating Problems

Anger-Releasing Strategies

Look for alternative ways to see the anger-producing event:

Did that person really mean to cut me off on the freeway? Did my child really mean to knock over my drink? Did my boss mean to interrupt me, or was he preoccupied with a deadline? Sometimes reacting with anger is the AESOP's first line of defense when defense isn't really needed because the trigger was actually unintentional. Ask yourself whether staying ticked-off is where you really want to be.

> "You can't shake hands with a clenched fist."
> *-Indira Gandhi*

Give yourself permission to walk away from the situation:

It's OK to say, "I'm starting to feel angry and I want to take a time-out," then be sure to do it! Learn to recognize the physical sensation you get when you're mad. It may be a pounding in your chest, rapid breathing, the surge of a headache. Identifying what you feel like when you are angry is a huge

Chapter 19 • Anger

step in anger management. Then, taking a time-out to go away from the situation and calm yourself helps you clear your head.

Create a stress-reducing environment:

Some time when you are not angry, pinpoint a quiet corner in your room, a sound-proofed area in the house, or an unused quiet space at the office as your safe space. You can also create this safe place in your mind and use visualization to bring calm to your mind and body. Research indicates that if you create a special, quiet

> "Each person you meet is in a specific stage of their life, a stage you may have passed or not yet reached; judging them by your standards and experience is therefore not only unfair, but could lead to unnecessary anger and frustration."
>
> -*Anonymous*

> "If you are patient in one moment of anger, you will escape a hundred days of sorrow."
> -*Chinese Proverb*

place or safe haven in your mind, both your body and mind will learn to calm down in that place. The key is to set this place up in advance so that you have a safe haven to go to when anger hits.

Immediate Action Techniques

By physically doing these suggestions that follow, you will change your body's chemistry by releasing your adrenaline surge.

These techniques address the biochemical imbalance associated with anger; they can work whether the anger is triggered by the situation, or just by your biochemistry. Think about trying some!

- Get the words "I've got to take five minutes" on the tip of your tongue for quick access when you're triggered.

- Pound a piece of scrap

wood with a hammer (no nails--too much control needed for those, and the object is not to hurt yourself!)

- Pound a red brick into pieces with a hammer, then sweep up the pieces. These pieces can be mulched into your garden and therefore recycled.

- Use the local batting cages, gym equipment, or handball courts as a focusing point for your anger, rather than your immediate peers or family.

- Have a stress ball close at hand that you can grip over and over while venting your anger.

- At the workplace, excuse yourself to walk the halls or get outside to circle the building a few times to regain composure.

- Grab a piece of paper and scribble out your feelings or draw a picture of your frustration. (This is a time when neatness doesn't count!)

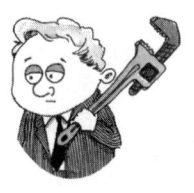

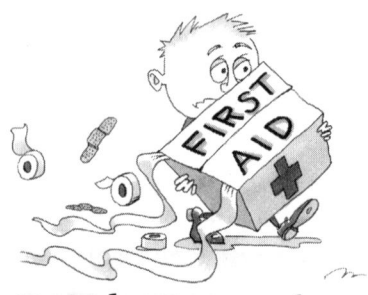

Need More First Aid?

If your life is stress-filled and anger is a common response, see:
Stress Reduction in Chapter 2.

If you get angry because you don't know what else to do, see:
Problem Solving in Chapter 3.

If anger is just one emotion in your many ups and downs, see:
Moods in Chapter 16.

If you have problems getting to sleep or winding down and this prevents getting enough rest to keep a lid on anger, see:
Sleep in Chapter 31.

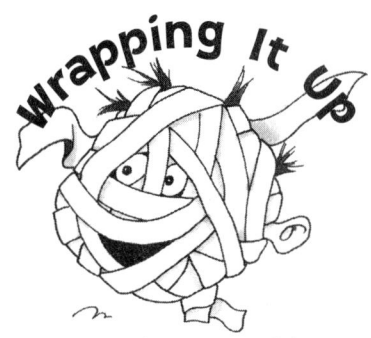

Wrapping It Up

- Anger is a normal human emotion. However, for many AESOPs, anger boils over and causes serious problems at home and at work.

- Anger and rage attacks may have a biochemical component.

- Managing anger can come from biochemical correction and/or identifying anger triggers and doing something to reduce them.

- Techniques for managing anger include self-monitoring, anger-releasing strategies, and immediate actions you can learn to quickly short-circuit an anger outburst.

> "The anger you're dealing with is as much a part of your SOP as any other difficulty you might be experiencing."
> *-Joan and Denise*

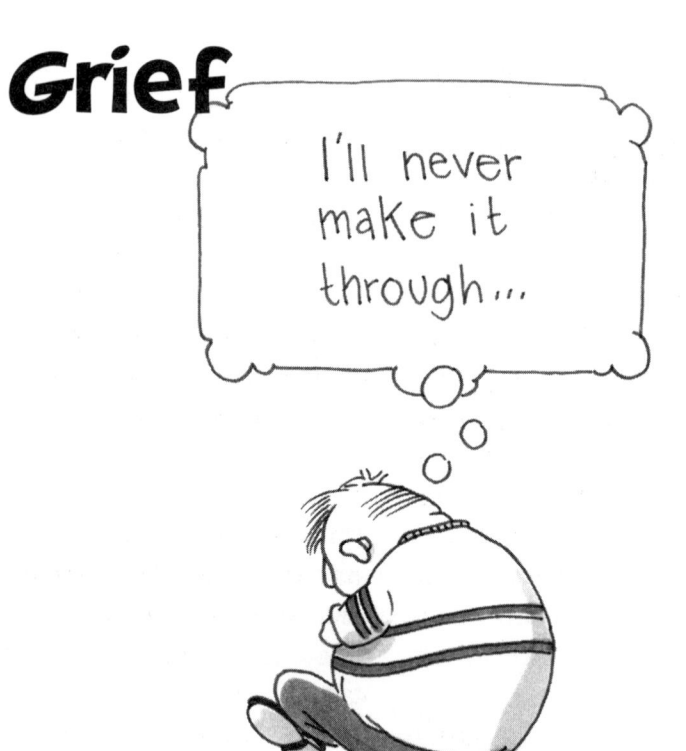

What You Need To Know

One of the least recognized or talked about aspects of being an Adult with SOP is the grief involved. This grief may take the form of a sick feeling in the pit of the stomach or a pervasive sadness that never seems to go away. There are many origins of grief for the Adult with SOP; often the first flash of grief is over what hasn't been accomplished in their lives, what potential wasn't realized. For the older AESOP, the grief may be even deeper, coming from the recognition that life truly could have been different but fearing that at this point there is less recovery time remaining to make changes.

Another source for grief is feeling that simply being an AESOP somehow marks us as not only different, but "less than" others without SOP. Many AESOPs have had a tougher time in school, or have been seen as a continual discipline problem; many have had teachers or parents say that they would never amount to anything. For these AESOPs

AESOP=Adults Experiencing Special Operating Problems

the grief comes from the hurt this has caused. Often there is deep grief for the hurt we have caused others by our words or actions, or lack thereof. And when there's a genetic component to the SOP, there is often grief on the part of the parents that they have passed their condition on to the next generation.

> "Regret for the things we did can be tempered by time; it is regret for the things we did not do that is inconsolable."
> -Sydney J. Harris

The Positive Spin

Grieving is a natural part of the life cycle. It's a valid emotion and merits attention and compassion while it is occurring. Think of your awareness of your SOP as opening a door to more fully understanding your life. With this understanding comes the ability to make changes, and with these changes, you can begin to accept your SOP and learn to deal with your grief.

Techniques

Honoring the Grief Cycle

Identify the causes of your grief:

As an AESOP, we often have unique circumstances that have caused us grief. Often there are multiple causes operating at one time. It is useful to identify your specific causes for grief before applying techniques to deal with them.

Be aware of the grief cycle. Know that you will pass through five basic stages of grief: Denial, Anger, Bargaining, Depression, and Acceptance. These can be experienced in random order and can be felt more than one time as you grieve a loss, but you will need to experience each stage in order to heal.

Set aside time:

The grief process and the ultimate healing must have time to occur. Remember that this is an important process and can't be crammed into bits and pieces of time while driving back and forth from work. It deserves solitude and space.

> "Allow time and space for grief. What one resists, persists."
> —*Life's Little Treasure Book On Wisdom*

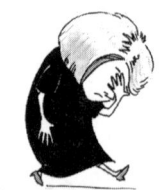

Be aware that family and friends may have grief cycles of their own:

Discord can occur as family members may be working through grief at different paces. At times, entire families can be out of sync in their individual grief processes. This, too, shall pass, especially if the family is communicating about their cycles. Be open with each other, and honor each individual's right to grieve.

Practical Steps for Grieving

Journal the grief:

There is a need to "let it all out." Journaling can be done by physically writing in a journal, pasting pictures in a journal, creating some form of art, or talking into a tape recorder. It is your choice whether this journaling remains a private chronicle of your passage through this time or if you share it with others.

Letter writing:

Letter writing can be another form of "letting it all out." You can write a compassionate letter to yourself as a child experiencing problems: offer love and support as an adult for the child within you. Letters can also be written to people in your past who have hurt you deeply because they didn't understand your SOP. Again, it is your choice whether this information remains private or is actually sent. If sending the letter has the potential to effect useful change, you may want to send it. If this process is more for your own healing, you may choose to keep it to yourself.

> "Everything in the universe has a purpose. There are no misfits, there are no freaks, there are no accidents. There are only things we don't understand."
>
> *-Marlo Morgan*

> "If we don't allow ourselves to feel the full range of emotion--deep joy and deep pain--we are less than who we can be." -Terry Tempest Williams

Letter writing #2:

Adults with SOP have often said or done things that hurt people. Writing a letter, making a phone call to apologize, and taking responsibility for the action can often be helpful in resolving grief you may have from causing grief to others.

Support groups:

Sharing thoughts and feelings often does a lot to resolve grief. Just having a sympathetic ear often speeds the healing process as we talk about what grief feels like and how we're dealing with it. Consider joining a support group of adults with your special operating problems.

Move ahead with life:

Recognize that identifying and dealing with your particular SOP can actually make it easier for you to move ahead with your life. For example, with an identified ADD diagnosis and medication you can successfully return to school, get that license you have always dreamed of, learn new skills or hobbies. Depending on your SOP, there may be accommodations available to help you in school and laws to help you in the business world.

Consider the impact of a diagnosis and treatment on your family:

Often difficulties faced by family members with SOP (including children) are seen in a new light when clearly identified. Treatment options which include counseling to deal with unique patterns of other family members is helpful. Once solutions come to the surface the grief can begin to be resolved.

Giving back:

Sometimes nothing beats being able to give back to the world. If you had a rough time in school, consider tutoring children with SOP. Your compassion for *their* difficulties as well as the knowledge of *their* learning quirks can make a huge difference in their lives and thereby in your own.

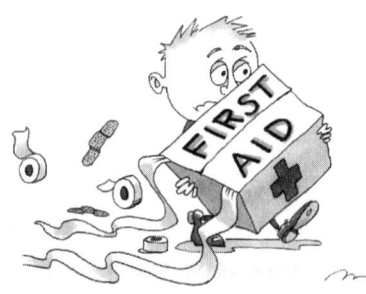

Need More First Aid?

If your grief just keeps hanging on, you may be struggling with a different problem. For help, see: **Depression in Chapter 17.**

If your grief is laced with **Shame and Guilt, see: Chapter 18.**

If you need a Higher Power or purpose to help you through your grief, see: **Spirituality in Chapter 34.**

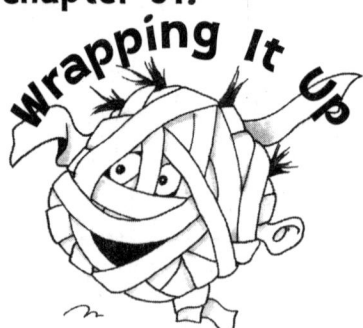

Wrapping It Up

- Grief is a very common

experience in the life of an AESOP.

- Grief may be felt for what hasn't been accomplished, what potential hasn't been fulfilled.

- Grief may also be felt for how we've treated ourselves as AESOPs, or things we have done or said to others that caused them grief.

- There may be grief in acknowledging the genetic transmission of the SOP to the next generation.

> *"Grief is a valid emotion and merits attention and compassion while it is occurring."*
> -Joan and Denise

- Specific techniques for resolving grief can help put it into perspective as a natural part of the life cycle.

Help For Yourself In A Relationship

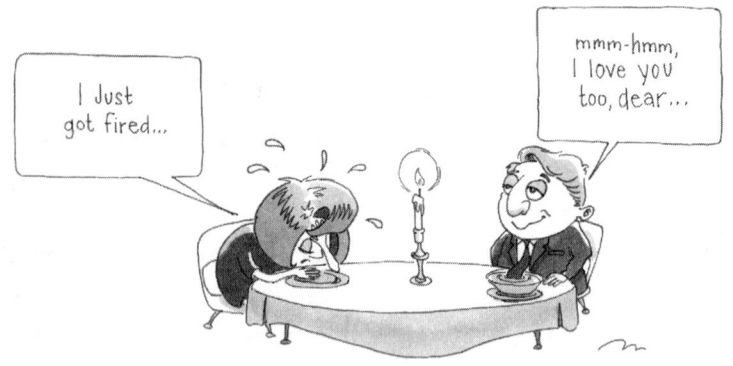

Chapter 21

What You Need To Know

"I'm really a good person; I'm really sensitive; I really try hard in my relationship. But it seems like everything I do or say is either misunderstood or wrong."

Relationships require work, and they can be difficult for everyone. But for the Adult with SOP, they may seem impossible. Having the words come out wrong, forgetting a birthday, giving up, blowing up, or retreating all chip away at the strength of a relationship. In many respects, an Adult with SOP is like a diamond hidden inside a chunk of coal, never recognized because of the rough exterior.

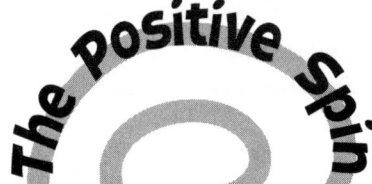

The Positive Spin

It's important for Adults with SOP to understand that even though our intentions may be absolutely pure, in truth our actions may be totally off the mark, rude, inconsiderate, and inattentive. We need to learn to

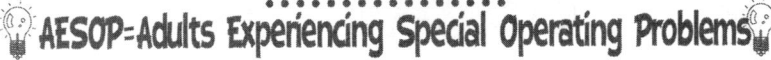

AESOP=Adults Experiencing Special Operating Problems

explain and clarify the things we can't change, such as our depth of sleep, and change other things that put our relationships in danger, such as coming home late or forgetting birthdays. Let's be honest; there are some things we can change about our behavior and some things we can't. Compassion for ourselves is a must.

Compassion for our partners is also a must; we need to recognize that, as AESOPs, we can truly be a pain in the behind!

Techniques
Increase Your Awareness
Identify your own SOP traits:

On a sheet of paper list all of your SOP traits, from your difficulty sleeping at night to your habit of blurting out comments without assessing the consequences. You may want to get feedback from your partner if you have difficulty seeing your traits for yourself.

Examine them one by one:

Decide which you cannot

> "Sacred partnership is a rich and deep friendship between equals that brings us sanctuary, soul growth and sizzle." -Sue Patton Thoele

change because they are truly biochemical in nature, such as your depth of sleep. Identify those characteristics that can be modified, softened, or changed, such as being continually late or blurting out inappropriate comments.

Maintain balance in your own life:

Realize that it is your responsibility to incorporate time for exercise, play, spirituality, and family time. It is not your spouse's job to be your keeper.

Recognize that your SOP traits may escalate:

Life presents us with many stresses. With the birth of a new baby, a move, or a job change, anticipate that your SOP traits will intensify. For example, if you are usually mildly forgetful, under stress, you could suddenly experience major memory problems.

AESOP=Adults Experiencing Special Operating Problems

> "The first love affair we need to consummate successfully is with ourselves, because only then will we be ready for relationships with others." —*Nathaniel Branden*

Tools to Build On

Work on communication:

Communicate clearly with your partner about your SOP profile. Discuss the traits that you cannot change and decide how they can be minimized. For example, if you have trouble waking up in the morning and typically hit the snooze alarm button four or five times, investigate using a vibrating alarm under your pillow.

Keep yourself out of trouble:

Be aware that a lot of SOP traits such as forgetfulness, impulsivity, or temper outbursts unintentionally communicate the message that you don't care about the other person.

Plan ahead:

Review your calendar. Buy birthday cards and anniversary

cards once or twice a year. Address cards, add stamps, and place them in your day-timer about one week ahead of the event as a cue to mail.

Call home and leave a message for yourself the minute the thought strikes you as a reminder about an engagement, anniversary, birthday, or dinner you have just remembered.

Call or email your partner during the day when you're thinking good thoughts about her to reinforce that you are. Otherwise, by the end of a long, busy day you may forget or be too exhausted to make the effort.

Before committing to an event, call your partner and check with her directly. Don't be tempted to say "I'm sure she'd love to go." Ask her!

> *"Get your priorities straight. No one ever said on his deathbed, 'Gee, if only I'd spent more time at the office.' "*
> —*Life's Little Treasure Book On Success*

Furthermore, don't call home to say "I'm bringing Sally, Ted, and Sam for a quick dinner; we'll be there in 30 minutes." Instead, ask privately whether that plan would be OK.

If you stop for a drink after work, set a timer so you'll leave and get home when you promised.

If you constantly run late, consider taking separate cars to a family function or to dinner at a friend's house so your lateness doesn't reflect on your partner.

Pad your ETA (estimated time of arrival) by 30 minutes, so you have more chance of being on time.

Be aware when you have overwhelmed your partner and give her space. At times, AESOPS can be too intense or too demanding. Learn when to back off.

Analyze your use of promises. Here again is a good intention which can really backfire. Develop the habit of keeping the promises you make--or keeping your mouth

> "Pick battles big enough to matter, small enough to win."
> *Jonathan Kozol*

shut. Before you promise someone reprints of pictures, think first about the six rolls of film that are lying undeveloped in your junk drawer. Will you really be able to follow through?

In society there are certain rules for politeness. If you abhor writing thank you notes, choose an alternative that will be socially acceptable such as making phone calls, sending email, or setting up lunch dates.

Be respectful of your partner's possessions and space. The nine coffee cups you have scattered all over the floor of your partner's car are not OK.

Prepare yourself for the inevitable relapse. No matter how hard you work on your relationship, there will be times when old habits creep in. Be alert to this as an AESOP pattern. Catch it early, change the pattern, but don't dwell on your relapse. Get back on track with your relationship.

AESOP=Adults Experiencing Special Operating Problems

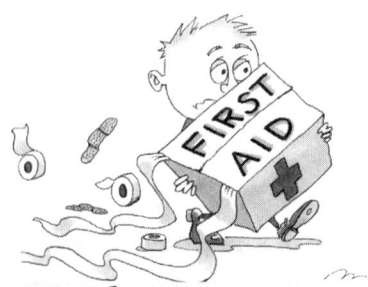

Need More First Aid?

If you're always saying and doing the wrong things in your relationship, see: **Foot-In-Mouth Syndrome in Chapter 15.**

If communication with your partner is a problem, see: **Intimacy in Chapter 23.**

If you're having problems juggling your life, see: **Balance in Life in Chapter 28**

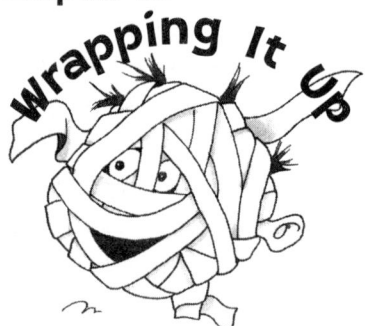

- Relationships can be both frustrating and rewarding.

- For the AESOP, they can sometimes seem impossible because of having to say or do the right things at the right times.

- Compassion for yourself and for your partner is a must.

- There are traits you can change and traits you can't.

- Identifying your traits, working on communication, keeping yourself out of trouble by using easy tips, and practicing relapse prevention will ensure better health in your relationships.

> "Let's be honest; there are some things we can change about our behavior and some things we can't. Compassion for ourselves is a must."
> *-Joan and Denise*

AESOP=Adults Experiencing Special Operating Problems

Help For Your Partner and Family

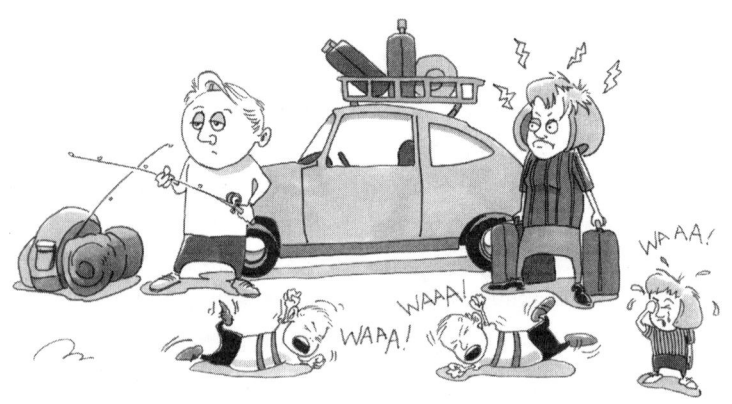

Chapter 22

What You Need To Know

Attention, AESOP! This chapter is designed for our non-AESOP partners and families. Please pass it on and read it yourself for some insights into AESOP/non-AESOP interactions.

Living with an AESOP partner can be terribly frustrating. Living in a family where both parents and kids have SOPs can be a zoo! (Ever consider, knives, guns, drowning?) In your relationship with your AESOP partner, do occasional fantasies of mayhem cross your mind? Do your kids drive you nuts with incomplete homework, temper tantrums, and endless demands for attention? Remember, there are fun, lovable SOP traits as well. Sometimes the trick is to find them when you think you're at the end of your rope.

Note: Although we've addressed this chapter to non-AESOP partners, here's something to consider: AESOPs often develop relationships with other AESOPs though the partner may exhibit different symptoms. For example,

AESOP=Adults Experiencing Special Operating Problems

one partner might be totally disorganized and live in a constant state of chaos while the other partner may be compulsively neat. Both may be AESOPs, but they can fall on opposite ends of the continuum. And one or both partners and their children may not be diagnosed. You might want to consider whether you and your partner fit this pattern.

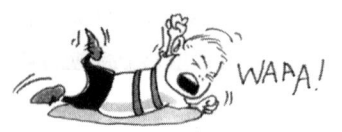

The Positive Spin

The first rule for the non-AESOP partner is "don't take it personally." When your AESOP partner blurts out "What did you do to your hair?" taking it personally can lead to anxiety or frustration: "Uh-oh, he/she doesn't like it." Whenever possible make the choice not to take it personally: "Wow, he/she noticed a difference." Remember, part of the AESOP's personality is determined by a genetic predisposition and body chemistry that is not likely to change. Other parts of the AESOP personality can be softened and modified. For example, AESOP partners can learn to take an adult time-out when tempers are flaring. You are certainly not wrong for expecting changes like this.

The first rule for parents of children with SOP is to identify the special problems your kids are having and to get help with gaining social skills, medication management, coordination with the school, and coordination at home. There's a lot of potential assistance out there, and you and your kids deserve to benefit from it.

And remember to look on the bright side! Where else are you going to find a partner or child who is so varied and so unpredictable that life is never dull? Who better to balance you as a partner if your own personality is stable,

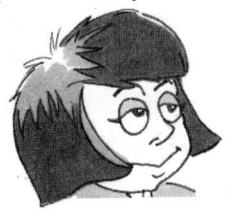

AESOP=Adults Experiencing Special Operating Problems

calm, and predictable? Who better to keep you stimulated in mind and body than your kids with SOP?

Techniques

Be Clear About Your Own Requirements

List your requirements:

Make a list of things you absolutely require in a relationship. Make a parallel list of things your partner is or does that drive you crazy.

Educate yourself:

Read up on the traits that are core to your partner's SOP and personality which are not likely to change. List those traits, then match that list to your list of your partner's irritating traits. By doing this, you are helping yourself gain understanding and acceptance of potential problem areas.

Recognize that traits may escalate:

Be aware that your partner's SOP characteristics may increase in intensity as life stresses increase, such as a new birth, a job change, or sleep deprivation.

Protect Yourself from Burn-Out

Balance your life:

Take clear responsibility for balancing your own life rather than counting on your AESOP partner to provide balance. Remember to take a bubble bath, go for a bike ride, put yourself in time-out.

Accept only your fair share of responsibility:

Decide how much is your fair share of responsibility in the relationship, and work at not over-functioning to compensate for your partner's deficiencies. If your typical tactic is to take over for your partner, realize that your anger at their inconsiderateness is bound to escalate. Moreover, as there are no consequences for their behavior, there is little hope that they will change.

> "We don't love qualities. We love a person; sometimes by reason of their defects as well as their qualities."
> -Jaques Maritain

AESOP=Adults Experiencing Special Operating Problems

This sounds like an easy solution; however, it often gets a little tricky. Certainly in some cases there are clean and simple consequences that can be applied and may shape your partner's behavior. For example, if your partner has agreed to do the grocery shopping, and it is not done, obviously there will be no food in the house. Take care of yourself by eating out with a friend or by visiting the local drive-thru. Don't bail your partner out by doing the grocery shopping yourself.

Unfortunately, in real life things are seldom as clean and simple as the example above. Let's look at another scenario. Let's say that your partner has agreed to clean both of the bathrooms in the house weekly, but doesn't live up to that commitment. This has been discussed between you, but nothing changes.

There is no way that you can ignore this situation because a dirty bathroom drives you crazy (but doesn't bother your partner at all). In addition, your mother-in-law (who talks freely to anyone who will listen) is coming for dinner and always checks the cleanliness level of the house. A possible solution is to hire a cleaning person to come on a weekly or bi-monthly basis who is to be paid out of a joint account, not your own personal income. With this tactic, the job gets done. If your partner feels that this is a needless expense, the expenditure itself will serve as a consequence and may eventually have your partner cleaning the bathrooms.

Identify your boundaries:

Be comfortable that you may need to stand your ground and enforce your boundaries. It's reasonable and healthy to request a phone call when your AESOP partner is going to be late, to have alone time for yourself, to set a bed time. Partners with SOP may resist these needs because they are not spontaneous or don't fit with their preconceived ideas. Stand firm!

Be Prepared to Negotiate Differences

Identify traits of your AESOP partner:

With all of us there are some

traits that are such an integral part of our personality that actual change is difficult. For example, your AESOP partner may have an extremely slow rate of thinking, talking, and moving. This trait may be genetically implanted in such a way that it cannot be changed, yet even though you realize this, it still drives you crazy. With these types of traits, negotiating a compromise may work. Try something like, "I know you are doing your best, but it still takes you forever to get across an idea. This is extremely difficult for me to deal with. What can we do to solve this?"

Once the problem is on the table, a suggested solution may be asking your partner to jot down a few notes to help organize the thought process. Another solution may involve you as a partner compensating by doing something with your hands such as sorting clothes, pulling weeds, or washing

> "When someone gets you down, don't give up on them."
> *-Dad*

dishes as you talk together to keep your mind off the slow pace.

Set Your Partner Up for Success

Use a master calendar:

Post a large appointment calendar for the entire household on the refrigerator with upcoming events written in colored ink. Remember, for the Adult with SOP, things need to be visible and visual. If it's out of sight, it's out of mind.

Write it down:

If you want something done, write it down. Beyond that, put the note somewhere, for example in the car, where it can't be missed as your spouse drives off.

Weekly meeting:

Insist on a brief weekly meeting to go over the master calendar for the coming week. Identify upcoming events for yourself or the kids, such as approaching birthdays and family obligations. At this time, agree on specifics: who will be picking up kids from an event, who will be picking up dry-cleaning or groceries on particularly busy days. Write the specifics on the calendar.

Be clear and specific:

Many AESOPs don't respond well to indirect cues. If something is important to you, give your partner clear and specific notice of its importance. For example, if you are taking a class and it is something you are not willing to miss for any reason, state this clearly; don't expect your AESOP partner to have registered the class' importance to you because you've talked enthusiastically about it. This is also fair warning, so if your partner blows it, they can expect a strong reaction.

Understand the difference between "AESOP Time" and "Real Time":

If you know your partner is constantly late, pad the time. If they say they'll be home at 6:00, in your mind make it 6:30. If the movie begins at 5:00, tell your partner that you need to be at the movie by 4:30.

> *"Of course it is possible to love a human being, if you don't know them too well."*
> —*Charles Bukowski*

Allow for the "Late Again" syndrome:

If your partner is holding you up, go ahead without them. Eat your dinner, go on to the party, trust that they will fend for themselves. Tell your partner in advance that you will do this, so they will understand the consequences of their lateness--and try to keep anger and blame out of the equation. (You're here? Great, we'll eat together. You're not? OK, I am going to go ahead.)

Set Up Your Family for Success

Establish family rituals:

Families with SOP work better with systems or rituals in place. These rituals should define much of what occurs on a day-to-day basis in a family. For example, everyone sits down at the table together for dinner three nights a week, whereas, Friday night's dinner is eaten picnic style on the floor in front of the T.V. Also be sure to establish bedtime rituals. For example, baths or showers are done by a particular hour and everyone is in bed. Stories are read for a half-hour before lights out. Be comfortable in knowing the rituals that you establish for your family can be unique and tailored to your own situations. They are important as they will become security blankets once adopted.

> "A family is a unit composed not only of children but of men, women, an occasional animal, and the common cold."
> -Ogden Nash

Reach for warmth and connection:

As a parent with an SOP family, recognize that the goal of family time is warmth and connection. Families with SOP require more innovation and flexibility than the so-called "normal" family. Don't be afraid to try something a little off beat. An example might be ending each day with a funny joke, a silly song, or a special hug, even if it's been a tough day for getting along with each other.

Parents with SOP and Kids with SOP:

Recognize that where there

are parents with SOP, there are likely to be children with SOP, with their own particular quirks and requirements. Plan for them, too. Coaching and family counseling can help.

Structure family outings carefully:

Mutually decide and commit to which of you will be making arrangements or reservations.

Develop a standard list of items that need to be packed. This list can serve as a quick reference and can be updated as the children grow. Make multiple copies of the list and file them in several places, such as under "vacations," "family records," and "things to do." Chances are you'll be able to retrieve at least one copy from one file or another when it is needed.

Mutually decide and commit to who packs the diapers, the car, the snacks.

Pack everything the night before; don't leave anything to be packed in the morning (even down to the toothbrushes). Last minute rushing can be a recipe for disaster.

Develop the habit of thinking, "If someone in the family

forgets something, we can buy it when we arrive." This cuts down on stress immensely.

Pad the time and communicate about it regularly. If you have train reservations at 10:00 AM, plan to arrive at 9:00. State the departure time frequently and with conviction so that everyone is on the same page.

Insist that your spouse concentrate only on the task ahead of them. Give them a list. Use firm good humor to help keep them on track and focused.

Establish a schedule and stick to it as closely as possible. Neither kids with SOP nor their parents do well with sudden shifts of routine.

Outings can be chaotic, especially if children are involved. As things disintegrate, as they often will, keep your cool. Tell yourself this is just one trip out of many, and resist the temptation to blow.

Remember, as stress and pressure mounts, the brain of the AESOP shuts down. Fall back on the old adage, "This, too, shall pass."

In the event of a real disaster (such as multiple temper tantrums just before going out the door), take a deep breath, step back, and don't take it personally. Make the event happen. Canceling the outing because of a temporary attitude problem (on the part of *any* family member) weakens the family. The goal is to grow as a family and not to be at the mercy of the characteristics of your AESOP spouse or children.

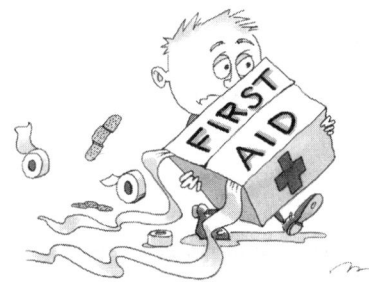

Need More First Aid?

If your partner or SOP family members have mood swings, can't seem to keep their minds off things that bring them down, or you seem to feel hopeless about family life, see: **Chapter 16 on Moods.**

AESOP=Adults Experiencing Special Operating Problems 304

If your partner's angry outbursts or rages are a problem you're trying to deal with, see: **Chapter 19 on Anger.**

If your relationship isn't flowing smoothly and the SOPs are getting in the way, see: **Chapter 21 Help for Yourself in a Relationship.**

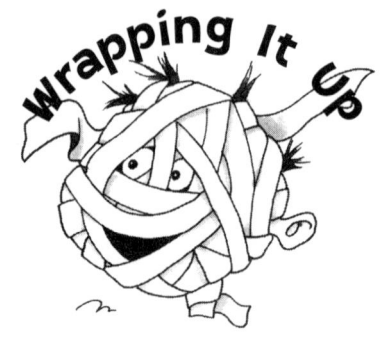

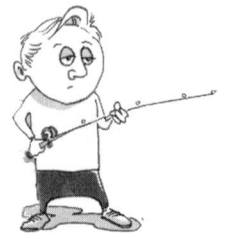

- Relationships are challenging anyway and can be especially challenging when Adults and Kids with SOP are involved.

- Often where there are AESOPs, there are likely to be children with SOP. Don't forget to factor in help for the kids, too.

Chapter 22 • Help For Partner & Family

- Body chemistry and personality style generate a great percentage of special operating problems. Be clear and honest about what can be changed and what cannot.

- Be open to the possibility of modifying behaviors wherever possible.

- Life is never boring in a relationship or family with SOP. It can be a wonderfully creative challenge.

- Techniques and tools to stay on track as a couple or family go a long way. Setting yourself, your AESOP partner, and your family up for the maximum success possible is the goal.

> "Where else are you going to find a partner or child who is so varied and so unpredictable that life is never dull?"
> *-Joan and Denise*

Intimacy

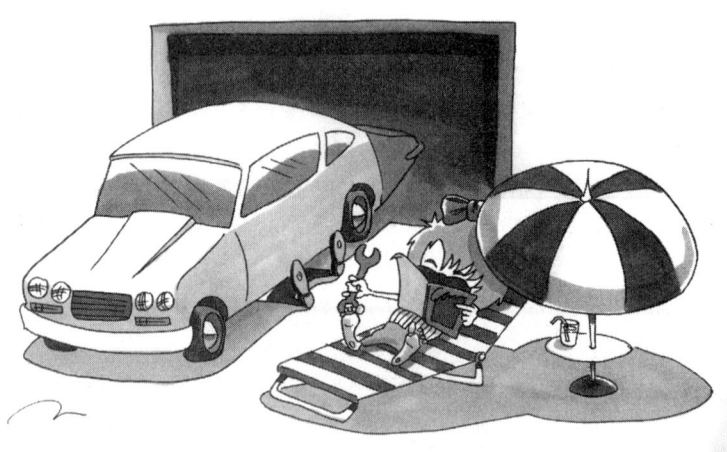

Chapter 23

What You Need To Know

The first thing that crosses peoples' minds when we talk about intimacy is sex. In fact, the word "intimacy" is often used as a code word for sex. While sex is important, what's even more important is real intimacy: the "in-to-me-see" that creates a soul connection. To visualize intimacy, think of a braid formed by the essence of two spirits coming together. The intertwining of the braid represents the intimacy of knowing someone at a deep and personal level. The doubling of the braid represents the strength found in two that cannot be found or felt in singleness. This is what we refer to as intimacy.

The Positive Spin

Most of us imagine that relationships blossom and grow with minimal effort. This is simply not true. For Adults with SOP, relationships require real work but at

 AESOP=Adults Experiencing Special Operating Problems

> "Trouble is a part of your life, and if you don't share it, you don't give the person who loves you enough chance to love you enough."
>
> *-Dinah Shore*

the same time provide wonderful rewards for doing it. Communication and understanding are the first building blocks that lead to the soul connection; they can then be brought to fulfillment in sex. Although intimacy may appear vague and mysterious, with understanding and specific actions it is obtainable. Once attained, it's a state so fulfilling, it's well worth the upkeep.

Techniques
Setting Up Success

Setting the stage:

Before launching into a dialogue with your partner to approach the subject of better communication and intimacy, ask if it is a convenient time to talk. If not, set a date for a mutually convenient time in the near future. For example, don't launch into a serious discussion when she's trying to juggle dinner preparations while breaking up a fight between the kids.

Limit distractions:

If the dogs are barking, the phone is ringing, or the Monday Night Football Game is in the third quarter, it's not going to be a good time to have an intimate conversation about anything.

Choose your method to connect/converse:

Do you communicate best by sitting in a quiet room with no distractions, or does walking together promote easier conversation? Do you like to touch the person you are talking with, or do you need a little bit of distance? What are your partner's preferences? Choose carefully for the best results, and don't forget to take the other person's needs into consideration.

Keep natural rhythms in mind:

Many people with SOP are night owls, at their best in the evening. These same people may not be able to put two words together in the morning. Sometimes, the rhythms are reversed, and the person who awakens chipper and ready to face the day may not even be able to put two words together by 9:00 PM. Choose your time to communicate carefully.

Allow enough time to tackle the topic:

If it's 7:15 in the morning and you have to leave for work at 7:30, this would not be the best time to bring up the subject of whether to have a second child or not. Do you get the picture? Instead, wait for a more opportune time, or if you feel an urgency to open the subject for communication, make an appointment for a later discussion.

Recognizing Typical Roadblocks and Developing Alternative Routes

Inattention/Distractibility:

If you've "set the stage" as we've suggested, and you're still having trouble, try these techniques:

- With distractibility, whether yours or your partners', hold the other person's hand as you talk to them--provided this

Chapter 23 • Intimacy

won't unduly distract them.

- Make direct eye contact whenever possible.
- If your habit is to speak too quickly, slow down.
- If you are overly verbal, condense your delivery.

Memory:

Remember that many Adults with SOP have problems in short and/or long-term memory as a core trait. These suggestions will help!

- Warm up for a conversation. Think it through in your head or write it down on paper to be sure you've got all of the pieces in order.
- Before starting a conversation, state your topic or question clearly; this way both of you know where the conversation's going.
- Remember that even a deep and meaningful conversation can evaporate. This can be caused by the chemical problems related to memory faced by many AESOPs and should not be taken personally.
- Be prepared to revisit previous conversations in order to

> "We should listen with one ear closed so that we can listen to ourselves, and the other ear open so that we can listen to each other."
> -Maria Suarez

start new ones with a mutual set of facts. For example, say "Do you remember the last time we talked? We were at odds about where we would go on our vacation. I'd like to pick that back up and offer a suggestion."

● If you don't remember something, be willing to own up to it. Bluffing can be an AESOP's quicksand; you can find yourself being sucked in deeper and deeper.

● If you make an agreement or promise, be sure to write it down and display it prominently for yourself. For example, write a note to yourself that says "Pick up Joey at 3:30." With an AESOP's typically poor memory, a promise is often forgotten. Remember, for AESOPs, if it's out of sight, it's out of mind. Any hope of intimacy will be decreased dramatically by forgetting to pick up your child at school!

Dealing with Long-Standing Patterns

Be careful about jumping from topic to topic:

If this is a habit, you may not be able to stop this from happening. You'll want a coping technique, such as a short list, to make sure you cover all the important topics; this can help you get back on track when you wander off.

Don't agree without hearing:

Don't just say "uh huh, uh huh" and commit yourself, without the foggiest idea of what you've just committed yourself to. It's much better to acknowledge that you're not in the best "brain space" to attend very well to the conversation, that intimacy is important to you, and that maybe you should take a raincheck.

If too much is coming at us, the tendency is to agree to anything our partner says just to get the noise to stop. The rule here is never agree just because you are flooded. When too much is coming at you, the tendency is to focus on just one part of the conversation or to feel so overwhelmed that the words all jumble together, and it's hard to track what's important. There are several possible solutions to this problem:

- Stop the person. Verbally clarify the main question for yourself, or if this feels impossible ask them to clarify it for you. If your memory's poor, you might have to write the main point or question down so you can organize and retain your ideas.

- Work out a deal that you'll use verbal markers or ask your partner to use verbal markers for what's important. During a conversation, state "this part is important." Next, lay out the meat of the conversation, and then state "this is where you (or I) need to make a decision" or "that's the most important part of what I had to say."

- Be aware that sometimes you may end the conversation because it's too painful or overwhelming for you at that time--this is a legitimate reason to postpone a conversation. If we blindly plunge ahead, sometimes we agree to do

Chapter 23 • Intimacy

something that can cause us far more pain or trouble in the future.

- Take shelter! If it's too painful to talk, take a walk, write it out, set up a later time to talk it out. Sometimes sleeping on it can be really helpful. Just be sure to give your partner a specific time that you'll get back to them, remembering that the goal is to deepen intimacy, not to practice avoidance.

Dealing with Hurt Feelings or Moodiness

Practice mental Aikido:

Aikido is an ancient form of martial art that deflects negative energy not by reacting, but by moving out of the way. If your partner is bombarding you with negative comments, imagine yourself stepping to one side and letting the issues or words move on past you. Realize, too, that your partner may just be blowing off steam. Do you really want to use your energy on this, or could it be better spent another way?

Don't take it personally:

You may be feeling like something's wrong between you and your partner when there isn't. Your partner may have run out the door without saying goodbye because she's really late, not because she's upset with you. Use the acronym FEAR: <u>F</u>alse <u>E</u>vidence <u>A</u>ppearing <u>R</u>eal as a reality check. Ask yourself: do I really have an issue here, or am I reacting to FEAR?

Take a time-out:

Write or talk to a non-judgmental friend, or meditate to get clear about your feelings and/or moods. It's much easier to communicate about them once you've identified them.

Be honest with yourself:

Is your body chemistry out of whack? Get yourself in balance before you attempt to engage in a conversation. Are you too hungry, too tired, too angry to talk? Are you in too much of a hurry to really focus on your partner? If you try to continue the conversation without attending to your own needs, you risk creating resentment further down the road. Honor yourself and your

Chapter 23 • Intimacy

partner with realistic assessments of how you're feeling.

Paying Attention to the Extroversion vs. Introversion Factors

Extroverts are energized by interacting with people; introverts are drained by interacting with people.

If you're an extrovert:

Realize you can wear your partner out and may need to give them space to be quiet and re-center themselves.

If you're an introvert and the conversation's just too much:

Don't be afraid to say "I've had all I can take for right now. I need some time to regroup." Don't judge yourself to be a bad person for wanting some time to yourself.

Problems Expressing Yourself

You may have legitimate difficulties with language that may be related to your SOP. In this section, solutions useful for multiple problems are grouped at the end.

AESOP=Adults Experiencing Special Operating Problems

> "Love doesn't sit there like a stone, it has to be made, like bread remade, all the time, made new."
>
> *-Ursula K. Le Guin*

Typical Problems Expressing Yourself

Be aware of your speed of processing. "Processing" is a word used to describe a person's ability to internalize and understand intellectual or emotional concepts. For some people, processing can take an hour; for others, it can range from several hours to several days. Some people take more time than others to process a conversation; some people are so quick to process that they get impatient with the other person for "thinking too slowly," They may even see the other person's slowness as a stalling technique.

What if you can't get the words out?

You may know what you want to say, but not be able to explain this in words that make sense, or you may not be able to find words at all.

What if you miss cues or hear unknown vocabulary?

Because of the inability to screen out distractions, you may miss a conversational cue indicating it is your turn, or you may try to fake it when unfamiliar words are used.

What if you don't know what your feelings are?

Many AESOPs have trouble understanding what we are feeling. Therefore, even attempting to express our feelings is much more difficult.

Solutions for Expressing Yourself

Write a script or use notes to prepare for your conversations ahead of time:

It can also help to rehearse a conversation aloud in front of a mirror or on tape. Physically saying the words and hearing your own delivery makes a difference.

Alert your conversation partner to your processing time:

Let them know if you process

slowly or you think so fast that you get ahead of yourself.

> "One of the oldest human needs is having someone to wonder where you are when you don't come home at night."
> —Margaret Mead

Use writing, thinking, talking, or meditating to clarify feelings before you start:

This will keep you from moving off track. Don't be afraid to say, "I need to think this through for a half an hour and get back to you," or "It helps if I make some notes as you're talking to refer to later; is that OK with you?"

Consider journal writing vs. talking aloud:

Sometimes corresponding back and forth through email or a journal can be easier than face-to-face conversation.

Know how to reopen communication:

It's okay to say "Remember that conversation we had yesterday? I'd like to reopen it because I had some more ideas. Would you be willing to do that?"

It's OK to state "I don't know what I feel" or "I don't know where to start":

This lets the other person know that you definitely want to communicate yet are just not sure how to begin.

Repeat back to the other person:

"Okay, so you're saying to me..." as a way of clarifying what's been stated up to that point.

Recognizing the Differences between Men and Women

Different things are important to each gender. This can cause misunderstandings. The following are six quick and easy hints for men and then another six for women.

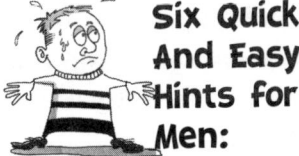

Six Quick And Easy Hints for Men:

- Listen ad Nauseum. Even if you think she's rambling, be willing to listen. Chatting is one of the ways women process information and connect with people important to them.
- Allow for decompression.

When your partner talks, don't interrupt. It's like getting past the foam to get to the beer. Women often need to go through a blow-by-blow description of the day before the significant issues even emerge.

- Remember her minutia. Things that may seem silly to you mean the world to her. Write down her birthday, your anniversary, be sure you know her favorite color, favorite flower, special coffee cup.

- Understand that small tokens mean the world. A card, a single flower, an "I love you," can be more touching than a dozen roses once a year.

- Provide for pampered comfort. If you're asking her to come and watch you play baseball or work on your car, make sure she's equipped with a comfortable chair, a blanket, and a book. She's likely to stay longer and be happier. Sorry, guys--you alone are not enough.

- Sex starts in her head. If you want a woman to be receptive to lovemaking, don't spring it on her. Planting thoughts and ideas throughout the day or week allow her to begin thinking about and anticipating sexual intimacy.

Six Quick and Easy Hints for Women:

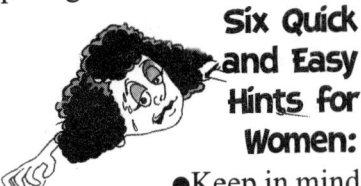

- Keep in mind he doesn't mean you harm. Men with SOP may do or say things that seem hurtful or off-the-wall and not even realize the impact. Be willing not to take it personally.

- Realize that his tools, car, and remote control are his territory. Men can be very territorial over certain things. When you try to clean up or be helpful, it often encroaches on his territory. Ask him first.

- Understand directness is a virtue. In the male world, blunt direct communication is promoted. If you don't really want to know how you look in that outfit, don't ask. If you want him to say something more flattering, you have to coach him.

- Remember he's evolved to solve. Since the beginning of human evolution, men have been the problem-solvers. If you don't want him to solve a problem you're sharing, you must let him know. Tell him clearly "I don't want or expect you to solve this, I just want to tell you about it."

- Be aware that men convert the phrase "I love you" into actions. For men, filling up the gas tank, maintaining your car, and keeping an insurance policy current say "I love you" in concrete ways. Learn to recognize the ways your partner says "I love you."

- Realize men sexualize affection; women affectionalize sex. Our culture encourages men to translate touch into a sexual green light. This is a big mistake. If a man wanted to jump into bed every time a woman touched him, a woman would end up not wanting to have anything to do with touch. Educate your partner to this difference between men and women. Being sensitive to this difference can make touching and connecting a less threatening, more pleasurable experience, which brings a couple closer together.

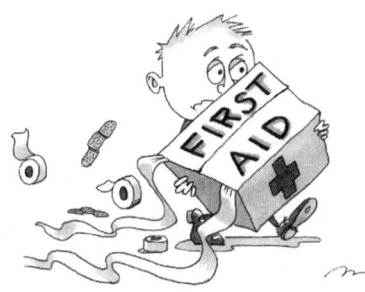

Need More First Aid?

Are you always saying the wrong thing? See:
Foot-in-Mouth-Syndrome, Chapter 15.

If relationships just don't work, see:
Help for Yourself in a Relationship, Chapter 21.

Is the problem with your partner or family? See:
Help for Your Partner and Family in a Relationship, Chapter 22.

If your sex life needs help, see:
Sex, Chapter 24.

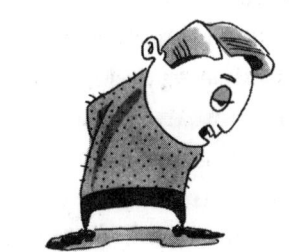

AESOP=Adults Experiencing Special Operating Problems

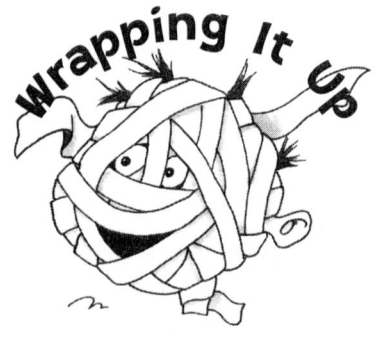

Wrapping It Up

- Intimacy isn't just sex; it's "in-to-me-see," a sharing, a closeness, a soul connection.

- Building intimacy requires two key components: strong communication skills and increasing your understanding of yourself and your partner.

- There are techniques for setting the stage to increase intimacy. These include limiting distractions, choosing how you will converse, taking natural body rhythms into account, and allowing enough time to tackle the topic.

- Inattention/distractibility, memory problems, old patterns, hurt feelings, moodiness, extroversion vs. introversion, and problems with self-expression can cause roadblocks to strengthening communication and building understanding.

- Recognizing variations in male and female styles of communicating helps improve intimacy.

- There are many solutions available to move us toward healthier, more fulfilling intimate relationships.

> "Although intimacy may appear vague and mysterious, with understanding and specific actions it is obtainable. Once attained, it's a state so fulfilling, it's well worth the upkeep."
> *-Joan and Denise*

AESOP=Adults Experiencing Special Operating Problems

Sex

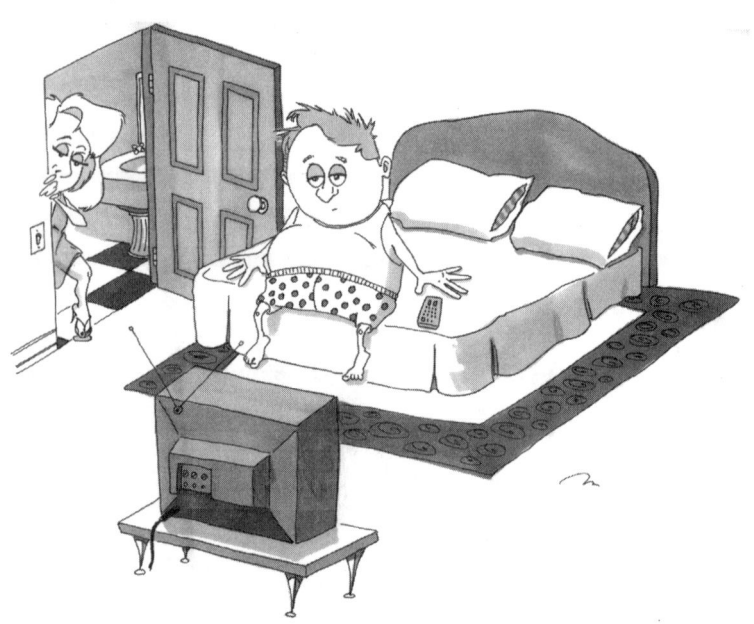

Chapter 24

What You Need To Know

AESOPs with their changeable body chemistries and varied traits often have problems with sex. AESOPs' complaints may range from "I can't concentrate on sex," to "I can't get my mind off sex," or "I just can't get the cues right."

A good sexual relationship has two aspects. One is the excitement that surrounds sex, and the other is a companionable, soft, feeling of comfort that is present with good sex. For all couples it takes effort to achieve a healthy sexual relationship including both of these aspects. It also takes effort to maintain this level of "good sex" through different phases of the relationship, which in some cases may span decades and encompass the full spectrum of life including the beginning of a relationship, children, the empty nest syndrome and death.

To make matters even more interesting, sex is perceived differently by males and females. For males in our culture there is a conflict. They

AESOP=Adults Experiencing Special Operating Problems

are conditioned by multi-media advertising to hone in on genital areas. However, they are still supposed to meet a woman's emotional needs for intimacy. For females, love begins in their heads and then moves to other parts of their bodies. It seems like nature's cruel joke that men can be ready for sex in two minutes, while women may need twenty-five minutes or more to get aroused. Because of these differences, partners in a relationship often begin to feel that their needs are not met or even understood. Worse, they may feel they are not "truly" loved by their partner.

We humans have greatly complicated the simple sexual act; it is amazing how many problems and deep hurts can result from misunderstandings surrounding sex. Sex is basic to all life forms; it ensures reproduction and survival of the species. With humans the same basic drive to reproduce is present, but the matter is complicated by two further components. One is that sex provides physical pleasure apart from the act of reproduction. The other is that sex is considered the cornerstone of a good relationship.

Very often it is not sex itself that causes a conflict but a combination of past history and individual traits that are misperceived as either a lack of interest or over-interest in sex. For example, the AESOP night owl who is ready for sex at 11:00 PM is crushed when he is rejected by his partner who is a morning person and most receptive to sex at 5:00 AM.

The Positive Spin

For AESOPs, maintaining a healthy sexual relationship may in truth be a little challenging. All the AESOPs' traits must be factored into the process. AESOPs may need to do a little more communicating around sexual issues, a little more experimenting before they find just the right combination. Once this is done, the rewards are incredibly sweet.

AESOP=Adults Experiencing Special Operating Problems

Characteristics/ Techniques

In this chapter, we have listed many AESOP characteristics that may cause sexual conflict. Then we've followed each characteristic with specific techniques.

AESOPs and Sex Drive Differences

AESOPs typically fall on one end of the continuum or the other in many categories. For example, they can be either hyperactive or hypoactive, depressed or rage-addicted. This polarity, which is obvious when we consider something as basic as activity level, is also true with sex drive. Because of their genetic makeup, many Adults with SOP fall at the end of the continuum where there is little interest in sex. At times when work or family life becomes chaotic, an AESOP's interest in sex may decline even further until it is nonexistent. Because of the emotionality surrounding this subject, the other partner typically emerges with hurt feelings and a deep fear that there is something wrong with them as a person or with the entire relationship. They have a difficult time recognizing that their partner's lack of interest in sex is potentially a biochemical problem. Predictably, hurt feelings and conflict in the relationship can be the result.

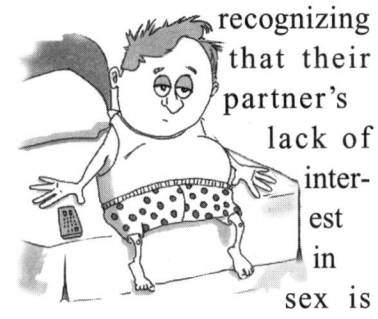

At the other end of the continuum are the Adults with SOP who find that sex and sexual fantasy occupy a great deal of their thoughts and are a major force in their lives. At times, this drive can only be satisfied by having sex several times a day, or in less extreme cases several times a week. A small percentage of this population may move into the realm of true sexual addiction. To the partner, this level of sexual need is often translated into a feeling that they are only an object used in the sexual act and not loved for themselves.

> "It's been so long since I made love I can't even remember who gets tied up."
> —*Joan Rivers*

Techniques

Communicate:

Be able to express your own feelings about sex. Understand your partner's feelings and needs around sex. It is important to talk about sex even if you or your partner find the discussion awkward.

Increase your awareness:

Understand your differences as they relate to the sexual continuum. Would you consider your sex drive to be below average, average, or above average? What about your partner's?

Compromise:

Sexual differences are very real. Compromise is the operative word for a healthy resolution.

Understand:

It is important not to just understand your differences in your head. Continue communicating, instead of closing down; this will allow understanding to reach your gut level. The key here is digesting what has been communicated.

Evaluate:

If sex drive differences are extreme and no compromise seems to be working, consider the possibility of a medical problem, such as clinical depression or hormonal imbalnce.

AESOPs and Body Rhythm Differences

Often AESOP couples have a night owl partnered with a true morning person. This gets in the way of both cuddly sex at night and sex in the morning before getting out of bed.

Techniques

Make an agreement:

Different arrangements work! The night owl can go to bed early, make love, and then get back up to roam around. The morning person can try setting the alarm early, making coffee for the partner, and helping them to wake up to get into sex. It's important to be aware of rhythm differences and look for creative opportunities to overcome them.

Restless Sleeper

The restless sleeper syndrome, complete with thrash-

AESOP=Adults Experiencing Special Operating Problems

ing and turning throughout the night, can have a negative impact on lovemaking and is actually much more serious than most people realize as it relates to sex. The partner may feel that the Adult with SOP is doing it on purpose (not true). The restless adult may feel their partner is just complaining over nothing because they themselves aren't aware of the extent of their thrashing. All they see is the pile of covers on the floor in the morning; they miss the bigger picture of how they landed there. Feeling resentful or irritated with your sleeping partner will almost inevitably carry over into your sexual life.

Techniques

Be aware of how much thrashing is going on:

Talk about it and recognize it as a problem.

Consult a sleep clinic in your area:

Rule out other problems such as sleep apnea or insomnia.

Consider buying a bed with two separate mattresses:

This will minimize your effect on your partner's sleep.

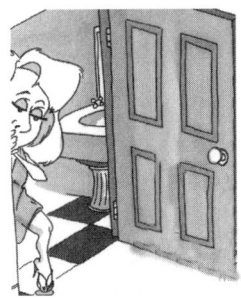

"Sex when you're married is like going to a 7-Eleven. There's not much variety, but at three in the morning it's always there."
-*Carol Leifer*

Cope with cover stealing:

Two separate mattresses on one frame may be made up separately to prevent "cover stealing" problems.

Consider totally separate beds in the same room:

This may be a useful arrangement, so you're still close by, but not disturbing your partner's sleep.

Implement a last resort:

Separate bedrooms may be the last resort, but not a "wrong move" for a couple. Making love in one room and then retiring for a good night's sleep in your own room can be a winning combination. To be effective, this solution must not be viewed as a punishment, but as a reprieve!

AESOP=Adults Experiencing Special Operating Problems

Filling The Day To The Brim

Adults with SOP often have just one more thing they need to accomplish. But where can sex fit in when the day's list never ends?

Techniques

Realize that healthy sex requires carving out the time and relaxing into the experience: trying to make love between bathing the dog and heading for the PTA meeting isn't an option.

Keep sex high on the list:

Many AESOPs' priorities shift and change all the time, and sex often drops to the bottom of the list. Make sure it stays near the top because it is one cornerstone of a healthy relationship.

Falling Short

Resentment over broken promises, unfulfilled requests, and old hurts can prevent interest in sex. Because of things they've either done or left undone, AESOPs may be perceived by their partners as uncaring.

Techniques

Look beyond the action:

If you have a partner with SOP, realize that often your partner may do or say things that hurt or insult you. These words or actions may come from missing a social cue or blurting something out without thinking. It's likely that your partner meant you no harm.

Be aware that forgiveness goes only so far:

You are the Adult with SOP and you haven't taken out the trash, finished painting that cupboard, or apologized for missing an anniversary. Realize you have to make an honest attempt to correct these problems or your spouse isn't going to want to have anything to do you.

Realize that sex is not a band-aid:

Hurtful things are done and are then expected to be healed by sex. It doesn't work that way! Issues should be solved so that sex can happen. If issues seem insurmountable,

> "He who looketh upon a woman loseth a fender."
> -Sign in Auto Repair Shop

seeking professional help might be a good idea.

Problems Reading Social Cues

For people with SOP, social cues are often difficult to interpret. Sexual cues are equally tricky. Subtle and not-so-subtle signals may be missed, leading to hurt feelings.

Techniques

Be direct:

Work on being comfortable enough to speak directly with your partner about your desire for sex. Practice saying "I'd like to make love with you tonight; how do you feel about that?" and don't take it personally if they want a raincheck.

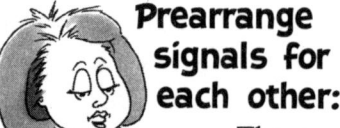

Prearrange signals for each other:

These indicate whether you are in a "yes," "no," or "neutral" mood about sex. Signals such as lighting a candle, laying out lingerie, or using a yes/no kitchen magnet work wonders.

Set the mood:

Use the phone, voice mail, or email to issue an invitation to your partner for a later sexual encounter. This plants the seed for sex and allows the anticipation to build.

> "The price of shallow sex may be a corresponding loss of capacity for deep love."
> -Shana Alexander

Feeling Overwhelmed, Misunderstood, Unappreciated

If at the moment or over the long term the relationship isn't going well, withholding sex can be seen as a weapon when it really is a form of shutting down for protection. Opening up to sexual intimacy when life isn't going well may be more than we can handle.

On the other hand, let's be honest. Humans often have ulterior motives, and there will be times in a relationship when sex *is* used as a weapon. Sometimes it can seem like the only way to get the other person's attention. If this is happening for you, you'd better have a look at what's causing each of you to go to such great lengths to be acknowledged.

Techniques

Use your head:

This is a time to take your thoughts out of your physical body and begin to use your head. Introspection is a way of looking into yourself to figure out what's upsetting you. It's also a way of looking at your partner with compassion to figure out why they might be pulling away.

Do a reality check on yourself:

Use objective people to check out your reality. Be sure to pick someone who won't just tell you what you want to hear. Be prepared to hear honest answers to some tough questions you need to ask: "Do I seem angry?" "Do I put my partner down?" "Am I rude?" By the way, doing a reality check on your partner is not a good idea because it's often seen as gathering votes for your side.

Communicate!

If you have trouble speaking directly with your partner, consider writing out or tape recording your thoughts and fears to share.

Plan a weekend away:

Getting away from family and work pressures often carves out a chunk of time so you can communicate and experience being together. If you do this and things get worse, move on to the next technique.

Don't underestimate the seriousness of sexual difficulty in a relationship:

If the above steps have failed, it's time to get professional help.

A therapist may even recommend a sexual "time out" to make space for more communication and the gradual reintroduction of sex and intimacy to your relationship.

Problems with Side Effects of Medication

Be aware that some of the medications used to treat Adults with SOP may effect your sex drive. Usually, psychostimulants such as Ritalin, Dexedrine, and Adderall and mood stabilizers such as Lithium, Depakote and Tegretol don't affect sex drive.

However, by increasing concentration or stabilizing the emotional state, they can bring more focus to sexual activity. Conversely, some of the antidepressants used to treat Adults with SOP (Prozac, Paxil, Zoloft, Luvox, Effexor) may carry sexual side effects such as a delayed ejaculation or inability to achieve orgasm. In addition, the tendency for AESOPs to self-medicate with alcohol (particularly if they have difficulty falling asleep) can impair or block sexual activity.

Techniques

Educate yourself:

Ask your doctor or pharmacist about the possible side effects of your medication/s. Even the little pamphlets that come with your prescriptions have a side effect section. This is important knowledge because it will prevent jumping to conclusions. Unfortunately, impulsivity can lead the Adult with SOP to think that there is a hidden message when there are problems with sex in the relationship. AESOPs may also fear they have some incurable disease, when it may just be a side effect of the medication.

Maintain open communication about the pros and cons of medication and sexuality:

For example, you might have the following dialogue with a partner, "We have to make a decision. My special operating problems include mood swings and rage attacks. Medication helps keep these under control but also decreases my sexual functioning. We may have to compromise between the strength and value of a long-term steady relationship as opposed to the more short-term effects of sex. I need to think about how to balance this out, and I want you to think about it, too. I'm willing to keep working with doses and techniques, and I want us to communicate openly about this."

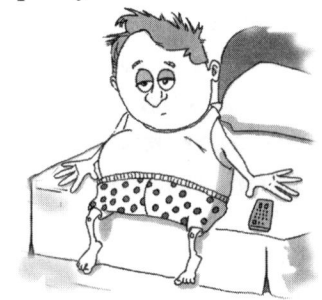

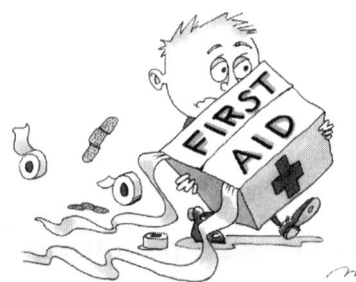

Need More First Aid?

If you need help in communicating better, see:
Help for Yourself in a Relationship in Chapter 21.

If you're not even sure what intimacy is, much less how to achieve it, see:
Intimacy in Chapter 23.

If you're too stressed out to make time for sex, see:
Stress Reduction in Chapter 2 and Balance in Life in Chapter 28.

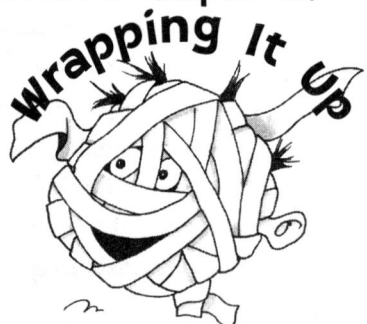

- Healthy sexuality is one of the cornerstones of a

good relationship.

- Problems with communication, body chemistry, and underlying resentments or concerns can interfere with a healthy sex life.

- There are certain AESOP characteristics or traits that can contribute to sexual difficulties.

- Certain medications used to treat special operating problems may affect sex drive.

- Open communication, negotiation, and sometimes professional help can make a huge difference.

> "AESOPs may need to do a little more communicating around sexual issues, a little more experimenting before they find just the right combination."
> -Joan and Denise

Problems at Work

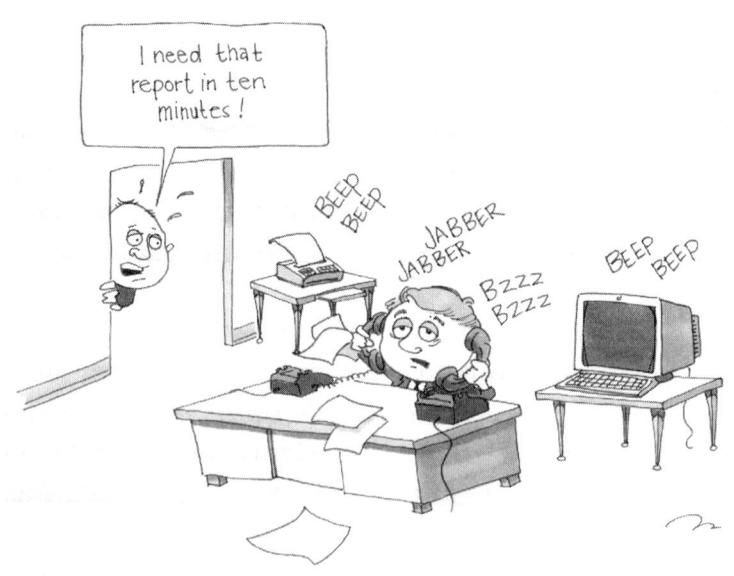

Chapter 25

What You Need To Know

AESOP traits can cause significant work difficulties, particularly in areas such as memory loss, inconsistency, absences or lateness, procrastination, and trouble starting and/or finishing projects. Adults with SOP may quit jobs due to boredom or frustration with the boss. We may have problems maintaining an even temper or keeping pace with expectations. Because of our AESOP natures, we need to approach our jobs with a plan in order to be successful.

The Positive Spin

Take a step back. Recognize that our unique natures make us very valuable employees. Our energy, creativity, sense of humor, as well as our slightly different way of looking at the world are all assets. These traits give us the ability to approach the demands of work with a fresh perspective. However, it is the mundane tasks that are

AESOP=Adults Experiencing Special Operating Problems

our nemesis. With those, get to know your own brand of SOP. Match it to your work responsibilities, and where there is a discrepancy, seek solutions. For every problem you encounter on the job as a person with SOP, you are capable of finding a workable solution. Don't give up!

Techniques

Gather Information

Research your job duties:

Consider asking your direct supervisor to discuss expectations with you. Talk to a trusted co-worker (who has the same position as you) for insights into the intricacies of the job.

Be specific:

Exactly what parts of your job are causing problems? For example, if your job requires soliciting business by phone, and you can't make yourself pick up the phone to make the first call, that is definitely a problem area. If your job requires adding columns of numbers, and you constantly lose your place, that is definitely a problem area. Use paper and pencil for this step. Make a list of the glitches. Then put them in a priority order. List the most problematic first.

> "You have brains in your head, and feet in your shoes. You can steer yourself any direction you choose."
> -Dr. Seuss

Brainstorm:

Brainstorming is actually a different technique than just listing problem areas (as noted above). Use your creative talents to brainstorm any and all solutions that have even a remote chance of working. In brainstorming the rules are that you must list any ideas at all, even if they seem totally silly and/or impossible. Often from these "far out" ideas something can be adapted or changed so that it will work and be a totally unique, creative solution. When brainstorming, using a partner often creates a synergism that allows more ideas to flow than you could possibly generate alone.

Identify the best possible solutions:

For example, if you're the AESOP who needs to solicit business by phone, you might write out a script to be used for the calls. Or, you might request a more private phone to limit distractions, or adjust your calling time to align with your peak periods. Each of these is considered a reasonable solution; try implementing them one at a time. After trying a solution or a series of solutions for a week or so, evaluate their usefulness. If they're not useful, move to the next one.

Consider trading tasks with co-workers:

You might find that your co-worker loves to do a certain job you hate. Renegotiating your duties could solve the problem; switching tasks may provide a helpful change for your co-worker as well.

> "Never, never, never, never give up."
> -Winston Churchill

Chapter 25 • Problems At Work

When You Approach Your Boss or Supervisor

Make a list:

Make a list (on paper) of your problem areas and proposed solutions. Make sure the list is clear and concise. You will be sharing this list with your boss or supervisor, so consider running it past one or two trusted people to make sure it makes sense and presents your ideas effectively.

Make an appointment:

Don't just drop in and expect your supervisor's complete attention. Ask if you can have 15 or 20 minutes of his or her time to explore some ideas. Make sure you ask for enough time to make your point(s). If you run out of time or your supervisor says he or she will think about it, ask how long you should wait before making a follow-up appointment.

Remember productivity first:

Remember that productivity is the primary goal in any profit-oriented business. Find ways to convince your employer that the changes or modifications you are proposing will boost business by increasing productivity. This is a valuable and effective selling point.

Does the Americans with Disabilities Act Apply in Your Case?

What is the ADA?

The ADA is a law designed to protect people with disabilities from discrimination in employment. It also ensures access to government services, and public accommodations.

Who is protected by the ADA?

The ADA protects people with both physical and emotional disabilities. For purposes of the ADA, a person is considered to be "disabled" if he or she has a physical or emotional impairment that substantially limits one or more of his or her major life activities.

It is important to realize that the ADA does not require you to tell your employer that you have any kind of a disability that may require accommodations prior to being hired. The law is also very specific and states that neither may the employer ask you in any way (even subtly) if you have a

> "The brain is a wonderful organ, it starts working the moment you get up in the morning and does not stop until you get to the office."
> *-Robert Frost*

disability or if you are on medication.

What kind of protection is provided?

The term to understand here is "reasonable accommodations." The ADA stipulates that reasonable accommodations are strategies such as job restructuring or reassignment, modified work schedules, or modifying equipment or training materials. For example, one ADD adult completed a training program in graphic arts and was hired by an engineering firm to work from 8:00 AM to 5:00 PM, the traditional work day. Once on the job, she realized that she was so distracted by the hustle and bustle of the office that she couldn't concentrate. Thus she was working until 8 or 9:00 PM to compensate. Her SOP included a high degree of dis-

AESOP=Adults Experiencing Special Operating Problems

tractibility and also problems with concentration. She decided to request an accommodation. She asked to begin her work day at noon. This gave her all afternoon to interact with the engineers and discuss their requirements. It also gave her the remainder of her day where, totally isolated, she was able to concentrate. This type of accommodation is a win-win for both sides.

How do I know if I qualify?

The first step is to make sure you have an accurate diagnosis of your SOP. The diagnosis must be made by a "qualified professional." For documentation, you will need a memo detailing your diagnosis on the professional's letterhead. Try to find a professional in your community who is not only capable of diagnosing your SOP, but is also familiar with the provisions of the ADA.

How do I get more information on the ADA?

There are a number of books written about the ADA, and information can also be found on the Internet. Federal agencies who administer the ADA will send pamphlets and other written information at your request.

The Department of Justice has a toll-free ADA Information Line. Call (800) 514-0301 (voice) or access the web site www.usdoj.gov

What can I expect from the ADA?

The jury is still out on this question. Originally, the hope was that the ADA would be an effective and easily-accessed law that would provide real protection in the workplace for people with disabilities. So far, summaries of recent court cases note only moderate success. At this time, the best approach is to go to your employer using some of the suggestions used in this chapter, and to understand the protection and reasonable accommodations offered by the ADA. Attempt to work closely with your employer to design specific accommodations.

The last resort:

If you have approached your boss or supervisor in a well thought out, practical way and they are still unwilling to work with you on accommodations, you may have little recourse but to consult an attorney regarding your particular case. Be sure that you research an attorney in your area who is familiar with the ADA and also with your own particular disability. This is often a formidable task in itself. At this time organizations such as CHAAD (Children and Adults with Attention Deficit Disorder) or TASK (Team of Advocates for Special Kids) may have referrals. The Vocational Rehabilitation office in your area may have referrals as well.

If You Approach Co-workers

Remember that honey draws more flies than vinegar:

If you decide to approach co-workers about your SOP, practice explaining or describing your SOP in the most approachable way. Saying "Sometimes I get so mad I could just kill Mr. X" will not be received as well as "Sometimes I get so overloaded I just need to take a break to clear my head." Which one would you respond to with more compassion? Be sure to keep your explanation as simple as possible. Rather than explaining your poor memory with a lengthy dialogue, a simple statement will get the message across: "I hope you don't mind if I take notes. What you are saying is so important, I don't want to forget a single point."

Watch your language:

Most people are unfamiliar with the terms often used to describe our SOP. Terms like "OCD" (Obsessive-Compulsive Disorder) "rage-disorder," and

> "The one important thing I have learned over the years is the difference between taking one's work seriously and taking one's self seriously. The first is imperative and the second is disastrous."
>
> -Dame Margot Fonteyn

"ADD" (Attention Deficit Disorder) may not be as useful as describing the difficulties you have in layperson's terms. Most people can relate to "Sometimes I have a one-track mind and I just can't change tasks easily," or "It's really hard for me to get back to my paperwork once I stop to answer the phone."

Be clear about your motives:

Do you want to increase understanding and cooperation? Do you want to engage your co-workers' empathy? Do you want to proactively work out the best system to maximize your area's productivity? Having your goal or motive clear will keep your conversation on track.

Beware of the sympathy-seeking game:

If you are sharing your SOP with your co-workers because you want them to feel sorry for you or take care of you, remember, this can quickly cause resentment and lack of respect. You want to convey that you are a hard-worker with SOP, not a worker who should be mollycoddled because of SOP.

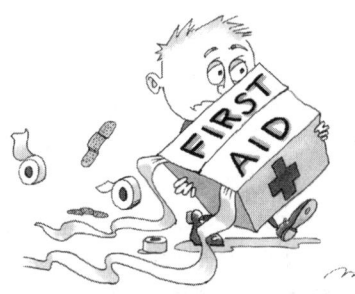

Need More First Aid?

If work problems feel overwhelming, look for ideas on reducing these feelings in:
Chapter 1 on Overwhelm.

If you are completely stressed out over your work problems, see:
Chapter 2 on Stress Reduction

If managing your time is your biggest challenge at work, see:
Time Management in Chapter 5.

If putting things off is a big problem for you at work, see:
Chapter 6 on Procrastination.

If you decide to use the Americans with Disabilities Act and ask for accommodations under the law, see: **Chapter 11 entitled Death, Taxes, and Other Necessary Evils.**

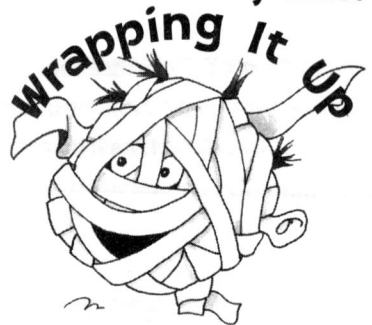

Wrapping It Up

- As an AESOP, you may experience problems at work because of your special traits.

- These problems can range from memory loss to always running late to quitting a job due to boredom or anger.

- You can help yourself by evaluating your job description and personal traits to determine compatibility, problem areas, and to implement a plan of action.

- There are strategies you can use to approach your boss or supervisor about your SOP.

- You may choose to approach your co-workers about your SOP. If so, take time to plan your conversation.

Chapter 25 • Problems At Work

- Often work problems can be resolved if we take the time to face them and plan out solutions, rather than hiding from them.

> "Take a step back. Recognize that our unique natures make us very valuable employees. Our energy, creativity, sense of humor, as well as our slightly different way of looking at the world are all assets."
> *-Joan and Denise*

AESOP=Adults Experiencing Special Operating Problems

Problems With Parenting

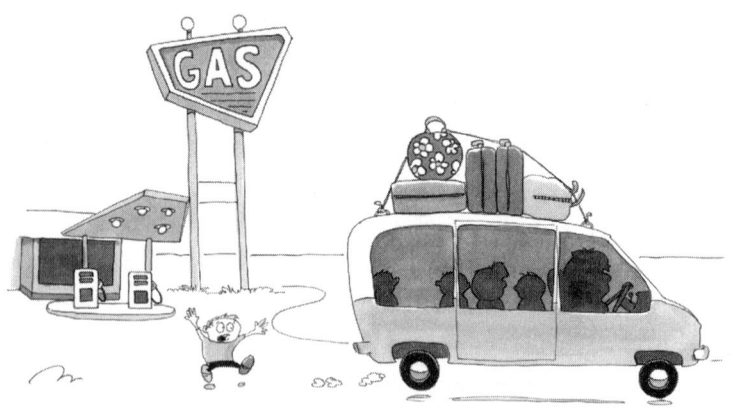

Chapter 26

What You Need To Know

AESOPs may approach parenting with some trepidation. We are usually well aware of our own problems with things such as inconsistency, procrastination, moods, and depression. Depending on the level of our own problems, we may feel that we have difficulty just existing in the world and are at the mercy of our patterns, with control being beyond our reach. If we can't handle or control our own lives, how can we possibly act as "responsible" parents to our children? Will we be able to help our own children with the nightly requirement of homework? Will our child's teacher spot us as unfit parents? Will we be able to manage our own work as well as the other obligations a parent encounters?

Another fear common to Adults with SOP is that, with all the obligations surrounding child rearing, there will be absolutely no time for ourselves. We may see ourselves as last on everyone's list. Magazines and the media tell

AESOP=Adults Experiencing Special Operating Problems

parents they must spend time (quality time) with their children. To have well-rounded children they must dutifully play Mozart tapes to them as infants and then hit the trail of Mommy and Me classes, Little League, and AYSO Soccer. AESOPs who have difficulty fitting in their own needs may wonder when can they fit in any sort of fun or a romantic relationship. If our AESOP is a single parent, that worry typically escalates.

> "I don't know any parents who look into the eyes of a newborn baby and say, 'How can we screw this kid up?'"
> -Russell Bishop

To complicate matters, traits that parents with SOP must fight on a daily basis are often magnified in the next generation--their own children. If the parents are slightly disorganized, the child may be hopelessly messy, turning everything they touch to chaos. When

AESOP parents, coping with a certain behavior in their own lives, try to correct the behavior in their child, it doesn't work very well!

Often children who are growing up to be AESOPs are truly difficult; parents may pass many sleepless nights wondering how their children will turn out as adults, and how they themselves will ever survive the parenting years. This combination of challenges can leave AESOP parents feeling a sense of desperation.

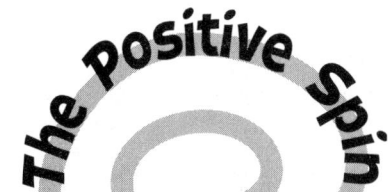

The Positive Spin

Raising children is one of the most important jobs we will ever have. It is also one of the most difficult jobs we can imagine.

Raising children is a constant process and often a constant struggle. Children come with their own unique personalities. Some of them are pliable, fit easily into the family, and are a joy. Some of them are strong-willed, determined, and a real pain to raise.

> "You give your children two things: you give them roots and you give them wings."
> -Anna Tochter

If your children have difficulties with SOP, the whole parenting process will have an added twist. As an Adult with SOP yourself, you are in a unique position. Who knows better than you what they're going through? This ability to empathize will let you be supportive and allow you to guide them along their own paths with the benefit of your own experiences.

As trite as it sounds, love really is the key to the entire parenting process. Children are given to us to nurture and help along the way. Your job in all of this is to love them and provide endless support. Beyond that, some-how deep in your heart you need to see their unique traits and wholeheartedly believe they will succeed. This mind-set somehow projects such a positive message that it creates the opportunity for real success.

Admittedly, this positive

mind frame is difficult to maintain through the day-to-day grind of dirty clothes on the floor and nasty notes from the teacher. Train yourself to look beyond the mundane into a "perfect concept" of your child's future. Once this is done, move back, know that you have done all you can, and allow your child to evolve into adulthood as a separate person who can understand and value his or her unique traits. Learn to trust yourself and your parenting.

Techniques
Special Note for Parents:

This chapter is meant to be a quick reference for parents. We have chosen to focus on special problems that children with SOP encounter. This is not an all encompassing parenting guide!

There are countless books written on parenting techniques. The problem is, with so many, how do you find the "right" book? How do you find the "right" approach? Here are some general tips.

If your child has been diagnosed with problems in a specific area such as ADD or OCD, ask the diagnostician or school counselor for books that talk about those disorders in basic, practical terms. (Check out bibliographies in the back of books related to those disorders for more references.)

Investigate a local support group related to those disorders. They often provide extensive reading lists and opportunities to learn from others living with the same SOP.

Realize that you may find bits and pieces of helpful techniques and advice in several books; don't expect one book to provide the whole answer.

Some authors are great for ideas about parenting small children, but are useless when it comes to adolescents. You may need a whole new set of parenting books when your child hits adolescence.

The advice given in any book must somehow feel right to you. No matter how famous the author, the approach and techniques must be consistent with your belief system.

Parenting Tips to Try

Keep it interesting:

Anything done with a child, particularly a child with SOP, must be kept fresh and lively. Whether it is getting them dressed in the morning or helping them with their homework, keep it new. Routine, although very important for a child's structure, is seen as dull and boring and may promote resistance. Behavior charts or star charts will work for only a short period of time before the format or the reward must be changed. Anticipate this pattern and prepare for it by having lots of alternatives ready.

There is a place for routine:

Even though routines may seem dull and boring, routines also make a child with SOP feel secure. If the routine is changed (and this includes even a fun night away at Grandma's or their room being rearranged) prepare them well in advance. In fact, give them two or three warnings that changes are coming so that they are prepared. If your kids panic at the thought of change, talk about their fears and feelings. Once you identify their worries, brainstorm about what they could do when the panic comes up--call home? Take a deep breath? Cuddle with you for five minutes?

What about school?

If your SOP child is having problems in school either academically or socially, research the laws and the school's role in testing for learning disabilities or ADD. Prepare yourself so you know how to approach the school, what you can request under the law, what the school district has in place to help, and what your child

> "A mother is neither cocky, nor proud, because she knows the school principal may call at any minute to report that her child has just driven a motorcycle through the gymnasium."
> -Mary Kay Blakely

needs in order to succeed.

Keep commands short:

Many children with SOP have a hard time remembering multiple commands. If you ask children to pick up their toys in the living room, make the bed, and clear the table, you will be lucky if any one of those demands is met. Keep it short, keep it simple, and know that you'll probably have to repeat the command anyway. Often children with SOP have to break their tunnel vision to hear even the shortest command.

Teach consequences, not punishment:

In order for children to learn to make better decisions, they need to understand the consequences of their actions. When parents punish children without making a logical connection between what they did and how to correct it, children learn to live in fear of punishment rather than learning to make good decisions. For example, if a child forgets to turn in homework at school each day, the logical consequence is to stay after school in study hall, or to have mandatory study time at home before playtime, or to lose recess. If you use a time-out at home or withhold dessert the child may have difficulty connecting those punishments to the behavior. As a result, that punishment would be less likely to teach the child to make good decisions about turning homework in on time.

> "I have found the best way to give advice to your children is to find out what they want and then advise them to do it." —*Harry S. Truman*

Tips on Sleep Problems

Trouble falling asleep:

This is a significant problem and something many children with SOP cannot control. Be sympathetic, and work with your child to find solutions. Try things such as a soothing CD at bedtime, a fan in the room (provides white noise), cookies and milk at bedtime, or a back rub. If these measures fail, consult a professional.

Sometimes medication is a needed last resort. Sleep deprivation is a very real problem.

Fears of the dark:

An SOP child may experience extreme fears of the dark actually caused by the effects of a biochemical imbalance. See this as a phase of childhood that will usually pass and allow a nightlight, a bathroom light to be kept burning, a favorite stuffed animal or the family dog in the bed for comfort. If these fears become excessive, body chemistry may be too far out of kilter to handle on your own. At this point, consult a professional.

Videos and Movies:

A child with SOP may be unusually fearful. Beware that even channel surfing between programs where a brief glimpse of blood or an accident scene is displayed may be enough to cause sleepless nights. Be extra vigilant.

Sleeping in parents' room:

Typically, this is strongly discouraged in parenting books. Each child is an individual, however, and for some, sleeping with Mom and Dad may be the best solution. As a parent, assess your child's level of fear before you make a decision. If your child is truly terrified of the night, allowing him or her to sleep in your bedroom in a sleeping bag on the floor or on a cot is not the worst thing in the world. However, it is OK to keep them out of your actual bed as they often kick and move during the night, disrupting everyone's sleep.

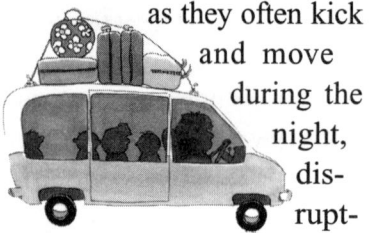

Tips on Stealing and Lying

Use a reality check technique:

As parents, many of us are horrified if our children steal and lie. This may cause us to over-react, even though the truth is that most children lie and steal at some point. To allow ourselves to put this behavior into perspective, we can check with other parents, read parenting books, or attend parenting classes. Once we have put the behavior into perspective for ourselves, we then need to provide appropri-

Chapter 26 • Problems With Parenting

ate consequences for each incident. We also need to work to remain consistent in our parenting strategies.

What to do about stealing:

Many children with SOP fight a continual battle with impulsivity; this accelerates in the adolescent years due to hormonal surges. This impulsivity often leads to picking up small items in stores and may move into full-fledged shoplifting. Be vigilant. If your child has sticky fingers, make sure that you are on top of the situation. The child needs to return the item to the store (or to the neighbor) and apologize. If this pattern continues, add time-outs or other consequences. Don't necessarily expect that once you correct this behavior it will disappear. Plan on monitoring for the behavior all the way through childhood and adolescence. Again, this tendency doesn't mean a lack of moral fiber in your child. But, still, it needs to be curbed not once, but again and again and again.

What to do about lies:

Many children with SOP lie

for what they consider to be very good reasons. Sometimes they lie to protect themselves, often because a parent or teacher has put them in a difficult position. For example, the child hits another youngster on the playground. The parents will inevitably ask "Why did you do that?" The child, not being able to say "I have a biochemical imbalance that limits my impulse control," will typically self-protect by saying, "I didn't do it. He hit me." The more the lie is challenged by the teacher or parent, the more firm the child becomes in his or her denial. The technique here is not to put your child in the position of being ASKED to lie. Say instead, "I have three children who saw you hit Johnny. This is unacceptable. Your consequence is apologizing to Johnny and a thirty minute time-out."

Another reason for lying is that children with SOP simply don't want to do something; this is often the beginning of the procrastination so common in Adults with SOP. One child who absolutely hated

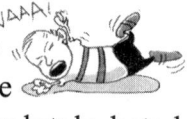

showers was instructed by his mother to take a shower. He went upstairs and quickly came down saying he had taken a shower, but his hair was dry. His mother took him into the bathroom and remarked that the shower was dry. He answered that he dried it off with his towel. She noticed that the towel was dry as well. His answer: "I dried it off with the hair dryer." Once again, the technique is not to put your child in the position of being able to lie. Tell them you'll be up in three minutes to see them soaped up and in the shower or that you will inspect them when they finish. Catch potential problem areas early.

Is lying a sign of a pathological disorder?

Parents fear that the lying done by children with SOP is a sign of a deep and disturbing personality disorder or perhaps even a warning sign of a future serial killer. Not so! Sometimes children lie to cover up not yet having done something; sometimes they lie to try to please their parents, and sometimes children just lie because things get dull, and they are impulsive. One first grade girl was bored in class; to liven up her life, she told her teacher that her mother was pregnant. This provided conversation during the year. After about nine months the teacher commented that the baby must be due soon. The first grader realized that she was trapped. She came to school the next day and told the teacher that the baby had died! The teacher called the mother to express her condolences and found that there never had been a baby. Parents are typically horrified with a story like this and are fearful that there is a deep sickness present in their child. Is this evidence of a pathological disorder? No; it relates much more to impulsivity and the need for excitement, followed by being cornered in the lie.

How to Keep Sane

Make time for yourself:

If you don't take care of yourself, you can't take care of anyone else. Parenting is a demanding, 24-hour-a-day job. Make sure you build in time for exercise, relaxation, and

> "Parenthood: that state of being better chaperoned than you were before marriage."
>
> *-Madeline Cox*

down time, and don't feel one bit guilty that the dishes are still in the sink.

Don't forget about romance:

Your spouse was there first. Make sure that you two have a night out alone. Make sure you have time to connect with each other. Use Grandma and Grandpa as babysitters and plan a weekend get-away.

Where is your mind?

Intellectual stimulation keeps us feeling alive. After a while, baby talk and words of one syllable just don't cut it. To keep your own gray matter exercised and stimulated take a class, attend a study group, or talk to a friend who has something interesting to say.

Surviving the adolescent years:

Typical adolescents still hold on tightly to their parents with one hand, and simultaneously push them away--usually by kicking them as hard as possible in the stomach. With an SOP adolescent this process is even more dramatic. Realize these years cause tremendous self-doubt in parents. During adolescence, there is absolutely no way to know if you have been successful as a parent. You certainly can't look to your offspring for clues. Stand firm. Keep constant with love, guidance, and consequences. Most of all, keep telling yourself that this period truly does pass.

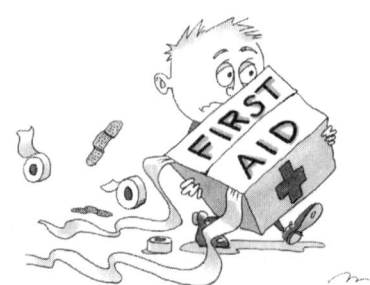

Need More First Aid?

If you are completely stressed out over your parenting problems, see:
Chapter 2 for tips on Stress Reduction.

If you have a hard time backing up what you say,

look up:
Consistency in Chapter 8.

If romance or sex is a problem in your relationship, see:
Sex in Chapter 24.

If you need more help understanding school problems, see:
Problems at School in Chapter 27.

If taking care of yourself first is difficult, see:
Balance in Life in Chapter 28.

If you need more information on the ranges of behavior associated with children with SOP, see:
Co-Occurring Conditions in Chapter 35.

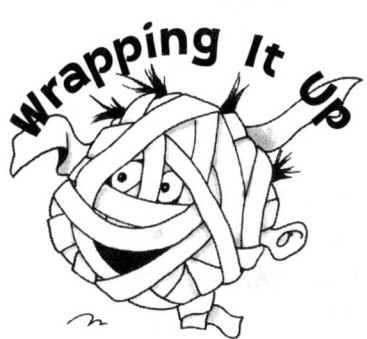

- AESOP parents approach parenting with an awareness of

their own personal shortcomings in life and a fear that they won't be able to do a good job.

●Beyond that, if they are barely coping with their own responsibilities in life, they question whether they will be able to add a whole new set of responsibilities and still have any time left over for themselves.

●To complicate matters AESOP parents often have children who also have SOP difficulties. In fact, many of the parents' own characteristics may be even more pronounced in the next generation.

●Raising children is a constant process and often a constant struggle. Children come with their own unique personalities. Some are an absolute joy, others are a real pain in the neck, and many are both!

●The best philosophy provides for constant love tempered with a realistic view of what is perfectly normal behavior and what is too far out.

Chapter 26 • Problems With Parenting

- Although there are hundreds of books written on the subject of parenting, some techniques just won't work on SOP children. Look for help from classes or books written specifically for parents of SOP children.

- Above all else, tell yourself frequently that children are given to us to love, support, and nurture. Our job is not to guide their destiny, but to provide structure and a safe place where they can grow. Ultimately, as individuals, they will each have the responsibility of finding their own path in life.

> **"Raising children is one of the most important jobs we will ever have. It is also one of the most difficult jobs we can imagine."**
> *-Joan and Denise*

Problems At School

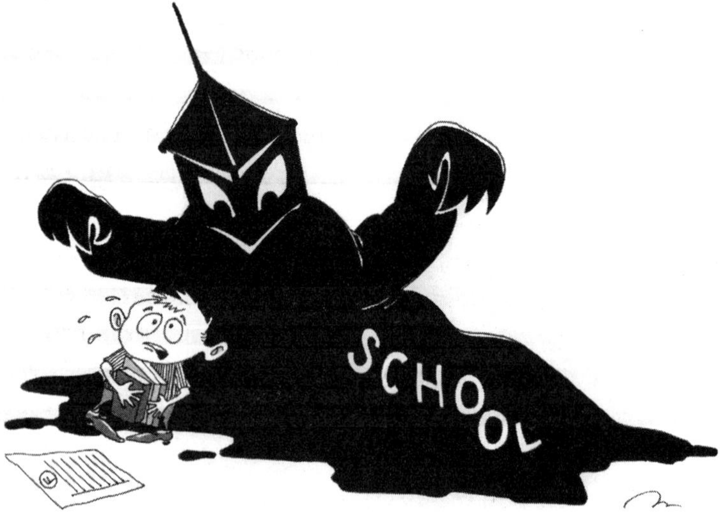

Chapter 27

What You Need To Know

For many AESOPs, school was tough; you may have lasting memories of failures in the classroom or angry confrontations with the school vice-principal. Even though you're an adult and you think you've left childhood memories far behind, this may not be true. Sometimes even walking through the school corridor to your child's parent-teacher conference evokes past feelings; that familiar smell unique to a school sets your stomach churning, and you have to resist the urge to bolt. But to be competitive in today's work place, you may need further training in the form of a certificate or an AA, BA, or MA degree. Even though the thought of going back to school may be daunting, it is important to realize that success in education is possible. There are many options, ranging from trade school and the community college system to a four-year university; you can also choose to be a part-time or a full-time student. If

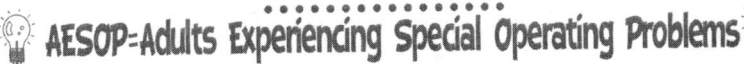

AESOP=Adults Experiencing Special Operating Problems

you are an AESOP with any type of learning problem such as a reading disability or Attention Deficit Disorder, help from the Disabled Student Services Center in the form of accommodations may be available. Replace the thought of school as a giant, insurmountable wall with a new, more positive image.

The Positive Spin

Although it may be hard to believe at this point, school can be a positive, successful, and even exciting experience. Realize that schools provide services to help you be successful. You have a right to an education; beyond that, you have a right to assistance to achieve that education. Our laws recognize that learning problems are very real, and they provide legal help to insure that learning disabilities will not be roadblocks to success.

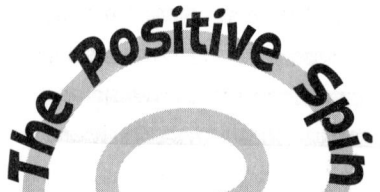

Techniques
Before You Enroll

Make a list of your school-related strengths and skills:

Be specific. Think about the positive images you have about returning to your education. Your strengths and skills list might begin: "I can understand anything if someone explains it to me." "I am a whiz at numbers." "I love to learn new things." " I am a good writer." This sets you up to recognize that you absolutely, positively, do have strengths.

Make a list of your school-related personal challenges and nightmares:

No matter how painful, it is important to dig down deep into your memories and be specific. For example, your list might begin: "I freeze on tests." "I can't concentrate for more than ten minutes at a time." "I transpose numbers on scantrons." "I have trouble getting assignments done on time." "In a test I am distracted by everything and can't think." Analyze your list and see if there is a pattern.

For example, many of the difficulties in the list above center around test-taking. Once a category is identified, it can be tackled and solved.

Consider your possible career choices:

Look in the Dictionary of Occupational Titles (DOT) at your local library for specific details of careers that might appeal to you. Compare your own strengths and weaknesses to the requirements of your career choice. Make sure the two are a match. For example, suppose a position selling pharmaceuticals to the medical industry excites your imagination. You've always loved to learn about new medical advances and the money is good. So far it seems to be a match. But did you consider that selling pharmaceuticals requires you to visit doctors' offices and also hospitals? All of a sudden you remember that you hate hospitals. The smell associated with them inevitably brings on an anxiety attack. This particular job might not be a match after all.

If you want to short-cut your search, it is possible to take one of several vocational interest inventories, such as the Career Assessment Inventory by Johansson, which will help you pinpoint vocational choices with less guesswork.

Check out schools and colleges:

Check your local bookstore or public library for reference materials that describe the colleges' resources. Make sure you're reading the most current material. Take advantage of information on the Internet and visit college sites by way of this electronic marvel.

Do even more homework:

Match the schools you are considering with your capabilities and career choice. Most schools have specific strengths and are known for their programs in particular areas such as architecture or teacher training. Make sure your plans and the school you

> "Courage is doing what you're afraid to do. There can be no courage unless you're scared."
> -Edward Rickenbacker

choose are compatible.

Is a Learning Disability or Attention Deficit Disorder Part of Your Learning Profile?

If you have been "officially identified":

If you have been in a Resource Specialist Program in high school or have been officially diagnosed with Attention Deficit Disorder, this enables you to check the box marked "learning disability" on the college application form.

Once you are enrolled, you will need to contact the Disabled Students Center on campus to register. It is not an automatic process. Be aware that colleges and universities are regulated by a different set of laws than high schools, so your previous eligibility won't automatically qualify you for accommodations at the college level. Additional tests or other verifications of your disability might be required. In fact, there are different and specific requirements you must meet to qualify as "learning disabled" as opposed to having

Chapter 27 • Problems At School

Attention Deficit Disorder.

If you suspect that you have a learning disability or Attention Deficit Disorder:

It is entirely possible that you have suffered from either one of these conditions and were never diagnosed. This can occur if you were one of those "easy," compliant kids who never caused problems in the classroom, or if your be-havior was so outrageous that you were branded a "discipline problem," or if you were very bright and school never presented a problem for you until you reached the college level. Ask yourself if you developed an intense dislike for school or if school seemed unusually difficult for you (even if your grades were acceptable). Comments from teachers often provide clues as well. Drag out your report cards from elementary school and high school.

Did teachers routinely make comments that you were "not working to your potential," that you were inattentive, or distracted in the classroom? Did they note that you had difficulty beginning or completing classroom assignments? Did you have an early diagnosis of some type of a learning disability that allowed you to be placed in "Special Education" or in a Resource Specialist Program?

If you feel it is important to pursue the possibility of either a learning disability or ADD, arrange for a private evaluation by a psychologist who specializes in this area. If money is tight, consider registering at a community college, and once register- ed, consider contacting their disability center for an assessment. (Insurance almost never covers an educational evaluation.)

> *"It's a damn poor mind that can think of only one way to spell a word."*
> *-Andrew Jackson*

Take a careful look at the Disabled Students Center:

If it is a possibility (or a certainty) that you will be asking for some type of assistance from the Disabled Students Center, make a personal visit

Chapter 27 • Problems At School

to the site. In a perfect world, services would be the same from institution to institution, as they are governed by the same laws. But this is not a perfect world. In truth, the expertise of personnel as well as the services will vary. As you speak to the Center's personnel you should begin to get a clear sense of their ability to help you personally in your search for education. Ask yourself, "Do I feel supported here?" If the vibes are wrong, follow your instincts and enroll at another school.

The Enrollment Process

Pay attention to deadlines for enrollment:

If you are enrolling at a four-year university, you will need high school transcripts as well as SAT scores. You will also need transcripts from any college courses you may already have taken. You will be required to take English and Math placement exams. This is routine for all colleges unless you have taken an equivalent course at a community college. Some campuses now accept applications through electronic filing. As you begin this process, keep a copy of *everything* as well as names of people you speak to and dates you receive information.

Oops, you have missed the deadline; what now?

Have a Plan B: realize that different schools have different time frames--quarters, trimesters, or semesters--and these often begin at different times. Consider enrolling in a nine week course just to get your feet wet and begin the process.

Once You Are Accepted

Immediately call for an appointment with an academic counselor:

Depending on the major or program you're entering, this person may be called the major department advisor or certificate advisor. The counselor will go over specific requirements for your major or certificate and help you set up your individual program.

Get it in writing:

Expect to receive a printed list of requirements that will detail the courses and their sequence.

Look for orientation lectures:

There may be orientations for new students given by the school, department, or programs. Ask about them, and plan to attend.

Visit the campus bookstore:

Take the list of course requirements and preview the textbooks for each class. Don't be intimidated by this step. Open the books in a semi-circle around you. Look them over. Make sure the workload looks doable.

What about your family?

Sit them down and front-load them about what you are facing. Enlist their help. Don't be afraid to ask a relative to help pick up the kids. You may need to hire additional help. The small amount of money is worth it! Remember, education will change the rest of your life.

Registering for Classes

Take a deep breath. Ask yourself:

Where will classes fit into your life? Consider your personal body rhythms, your work schedule, and your kids' schedules.

Would a class on study skills help you to fine-tune your study habits?

What about early registration? (Check with Disabled Students Center.)

Who can you talk with to get information on instructors who are approachable and sympathetic to adults with disabilities?

Registration is usually done by phone:

Fill out a worksheet (provided by the school) with all course numbers and times penciled in before you call.

Always have a Plan B with alternate courses and/or times.

If all of the courses you need are full, return to your advisor for help. There may be alternative courses you haven't considered, or there may also be a waiting list your advisor could put you on.

Now You Are in Class

Give yourself the first week to get a feel for the instructor and the workload:

If you haven't yet registered with the Disabled Students Center, now is the time.

> "The first time many of us realize that a little learning is a dangerous thing is when we bring home a poor report card."
> -*20,000 Quotes and Quotations*

Ask yourself honestly if you might need special assistance or accommodations:

Students often wait until they know they are in trouble before seeking this sort of help. This is a mistake. Set the process in motion early.

Plan to attend each and every class:

Instructors take a dim view of absences--particularly if you are asking for special consideration.

Visit instructors during office hours:

Let them know you are serious and determined to succeed, but that you have a disability. Be specific about your problems and offer possible solutions, i.e. "I have trouble understanding printed information, so I'll be using books on tape." "I have trouble taking notes during a lecture, and I'd like to use a tape recorder. Is that OK with you?"

Instructors are generally good people who want you to succeed. Help them to understand that you are serious about your education. At the college level, instructors have a great deal of influence over special assistance, so plan on developing a positive relationship with them. For example, if you are requesting extended time on an exam, the instructor has a great deal to say about the length of time that is allowed. The instructor can also make it much easier for you by making sure that the testing material is at the Disabled Students Center on time. However, the instructor can also throw up roadblocks that can be irritating and time-consuming to overcome.

Typical Accommodations

"Accommodations" is the legal terminology in the Rehabilitation Act of 1973

(504 Law), and it is also used by colleges and universities. It simply means that a student has the right to have a learning disability "accommodated" so that you are not discriminated against in the educational environment. To make it simple: a person in a wheelchair can't walk upstairs and is "accommodated" by a wheelchair ramp. A student whose disability is in written language, which prevents him from taking notes in a lecture class, is "accommodated" by using a note taker in the lecture.

To qualify for accommodations you must officially register with the Disabled Students Center. Typical accommodations follow.

Tutoring:

Tutoring is often suggested by the Disabled Students Center and provided at a tutoring center on campus at no charge. At times, the level of tutoring offered may not be sufficient, and you may want to supplement it by hiring your own tutor for particularly difficult classes.

Note takers in class:

The Disabled Students Center will pay a student in your class to take notes for you. You may be asked to approach someone in your class if the Center does not have someone available immediately.

Accommodations for exams:

One of the most typical accommodations is extended time, which ranges from time and a half to double time. (Requesting unlimited time is a possibility, although your disability must be extreme to qualify for this.) The second most common accommodation is test-taking in a distraction-free setting, usually the Disabled Students Center.

Using a tape recorder:

If you have a severe written language disability you may tape record lectures and either listen to them again or have them transcribed. Although most professors are willing to allow this, you must ask their permission as a matter of protocol.

Chapter 27 • Problems At School

Extended or modified time on the due dates of assignments:

This is considered over and above typical accommodations and should be used prudently and with explanation. If you have two research papers due in the same week, both of which require extensive rough drafts and typing, request a specific time frame extension, such as an extra week or staggered dates. Once this is granted, don't forget to thank the professor for his or her willingness to accommodate your disability.

If reading comprehension is a problem:

You may benefit from hearing the textbooks read aloud if you have problems with reading comprehension. If so, you can request services from Recordings for the Blind through the Disabled Students Center.

This service provides textbooks on tape. There is no charge, but it typically takes six weeks to complete the process, so get started early.

What to Do if Problems Start to Surface

Be clear about the problems you are having:

Identify whether they are academic, work-related, or personal.

For example, your last test score was an "F." Identify the reason. Was it that:

- You couldn't understand the material?
- You had to work a double shift the day before the exam and couldn't study?
- You have too many classes and can't keep the information straight?
- You caught the flu for the fourth time this year and can't seem to catch up on your studying?
- Your partner threatened to leave you because you're spending too much time in school, and you are devastated?

Whatever the reasons, break them down into possible solutions. For example:

- See the instructor (during office hours) about the test. Ask for help in identifying whether you need more work on basic concepts or need to back up to a more basic text for information. Would a study group help? Do you need private tutoring?

> "Many of life's failures are people who did not realize how close they were to success when they gave up." -*Thomas Edison*

● Speak to your employer. If you are stressed out about a pending research paper that is looming on the horizon or class requirements in general, your concentration may be suffering at work. If this is the case, a proactive approach is best. Be up front with your employer. Let your employer know that you are aware of the problem and, more importantly, that you are taking steps to correct the situation. Saying something like, "I know I haven't been at my best, but I'm turning in my research paper tomorrow and will be back on track" often does the trick. If the situation is more complicated and comes from biting off more than you can chew, you may need to make a hard decision and let your employer know you are planning to drop a class.

- Talk to your instructor about work. If unexpected duties at work are interfering with class attendance or your ability to study, visit your instructor during office hours. Explain the situation. If you need extra time on an assignment or paper, be clear and specific in your request. For example, you might say, "I'll be working overtime next week. Could I have an extra week on the research paper?"

- Do you need to drop a class, or re-organize how you study by using a study group or a tutor? If you are considering dropping a class, it is wise to check with your advisor first.

- Stress (as well as lack of sleep) definitely can damage your immune system. Do you have too much on your plate? Check out your balance in life: what about diet, level of exercise, vitamins?

- Reassure your partner that the courses will soon be over, and then you can give more time to the relationship. Consider enlisting a relative to help with the chores or the kids, or hire help.

● Check out your time management skills; maybe it's possible to free up more time. Would counseling help?

Help! I'm Going Down the Tubes

Think damage control:

The tendency is to run. Don't do it! If you simply stop going to class, your GPA will drop to such a low that you'll need to re-apply to the school and also request that your semester be erased. Instead, be proactive. There is a specific process for withdrawing that is relatively easy.

Pick up withdrawal forms from the Records Office and get the required signatures, usually from the instructor and the chairperson.

While there are deadlines for withdrawing, there are exceptions for medical reasons (which would include illness caused by stress). If you are requesting such an exception, you will probably need a physician's signature.

Even though withdrawing

from your classes may be hard to face, cleaning up a messy transcript from your past is much more complicated and time-consuming.

Know that you can start again the following term (maybe with a lighter load) and be successful.

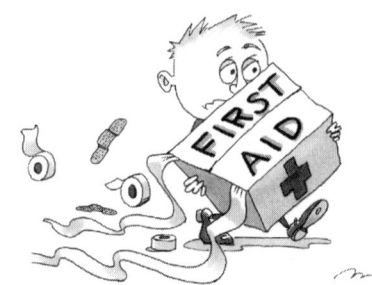

Need More First Aid?

If you feel totally overloaded, see:
Stress Reduction in Chapter 2.

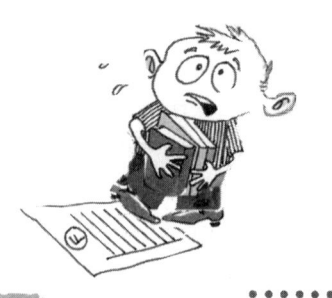

If you find you can't even begin the process, see:
Procrastination in

Chapter 6.

If it feels as though all you do is work and go to school with absolutely no time for yourself, see:
Balance in Life in Chapter 28.

If you have learning problems, but you are also faced with obsessions, compulsions or depression, see:
Chapter 35 on Co-Occurring Conditions.

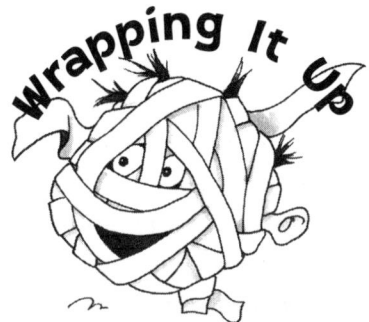
Wrapping It Up

●Many AESOPs have had extremely negative experiences in school.

●In today's job market it is often necessary to return to school. You may obtain a certificate of proficiency, or an AA, BA or MA degree to qualify for a new job or gain

AESOP=Adults Experiencing Special Operating Problems

advancement in a long-standing job.

●With federal regulations regarding learning disabilities as well as ADD, you can expect the re-entry process to be much easier than you ever anticipated.

●When you're ready to enroll, you may be eligible for special enrollment procedures by registering through the Disabled Students Center.

●When you're in a class, there are many different avenues available to put success within your grasp.

●The key is developing an understanding of your own learning glitches and combining that knowledge with information about special services that are available to you. You can be successful! Get to work!

> "Sometimes even walking through the school corridor to your child's parent-teacher conference evokes past feelings; that familiar smell unique to a school sets your stomach churning, and you have to resist the urge to bolt."
>
> *-Joan and Denise*

Balance In Life

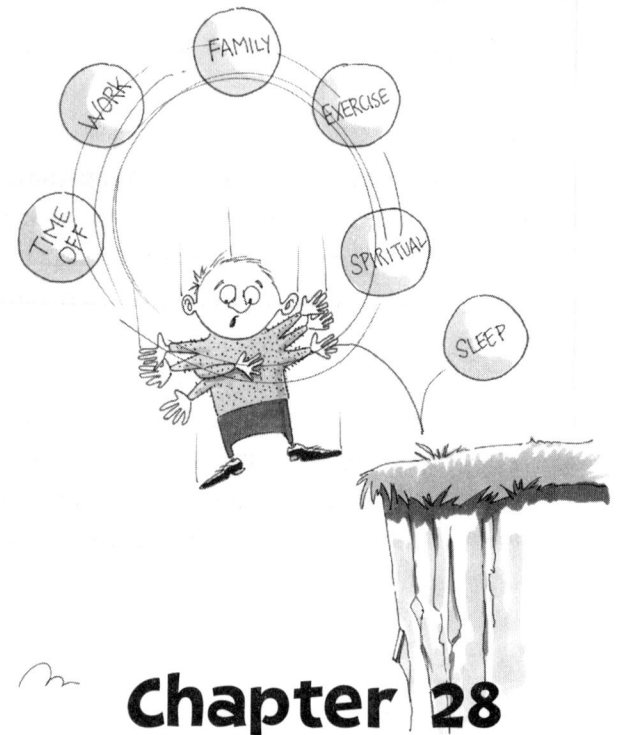

Chapter 28

What You Need To Know

An old Chinese proverb states that life's ideal balance is eight hours of work, eight hours of leisure and eight hours of sleep. This may be an "ideal," but let's be honest; Adults with SOP typically operate with a different reality structure. This reality structure encompasses a wider definition of balance. Think of life as a continuum: normal is in the middle, while Adults with SOP typically operate at either end of the continuum, moving through brief periods of normalcy as they travel from one end of the continuum to the other. However, they have difficulty doing anything in moderation. They also have problems maintaining any type of consistency over time. For some AESOPs, balance is achieved by intervals. They work hard and focus totally for a period of time. This represents one end of the continuum. Then they regroup and play or vacation or crash for a period of time. This represents the other end of the continuum. In this way

AESOP=Adults Experiencing Special Operating Problems

they do manage some sort of an overall balance in life, a balance achieved in a unique but workable manner.

> "Each day and the living of it, has to be a conscious creation in which discipline and order are relieved with some play and some pure foolishness."
>
> *-May Sarton*

Problems can often occur in relationships because a partner doesn't understand the AESOP's unique approach to balance. It takes time and effort to bring your partner into the loop.

Problems also occur when the Adult with SOP goes beyond the edges of the continuum. AESOPs are prone to extremes of "way too much" or "nothing at all." At these points on the scale, things move into the area of obsessions and can be disastrous. For example, an AESOP who exercises relentlessly to the

Chapter 28 • Balance In Life

point of torn muscles or ignoring other basics in life has gone off the scale and is out of balance. Internet addiction also ranks at this level. On the other end of the spectrum, feeling totally immobilized or "burned out" is an example of the "nothing at all" response. This person may have serious trouble getting out of bed, much less getting to work every day.

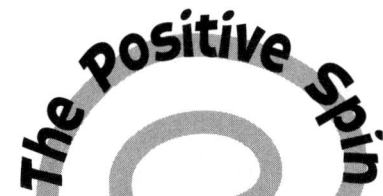

The Positive Spin

Realize that it is the nature of the Adult with SOP to move from one end of the continuum to the other, experiencing only brief periods of what might be considered normal. With their need for zest and creativity, AESOPs must be able to understand their travels along the continuum and embrace the necessity for this pattern in life and the possible flashes of brilliance and heightened productivity during the upswing. However, they must also be alert for the danger when the extremes become too pronounced. Remember, magazine articles and talk shows that encourage balance and moderation in a traditional manner may not work for the Adult with SOP.

> "The trouble with using experience as a guide is that the final exam often comes first and then the lesson."
> *-Unknown*

Techniques

Recognize your pattern:

Identify the periods of time you spend being totally focused and putting in long hours immersed in work or in a project. Make sure that you allow for the other end of the continuum: a balancing period of down-time or decompression.

Bring your partner into the loop:

Living with an AESOP can be a challenge. The entire concept of peak periods of performance balanced by down-time is foreign to a non-AESOP. Make sure that you can explain your strategies for achieving balance to your partner. Then, negotiate with your partner to make sure that your unique methods of achieving balance are OK with them.

Plan ahead:

Use a master calendar to predict peak periods of work or stress in your life that will need to be counterbalanced with some down-time or a weekend out of town. Be careful not to over-schedule peak periods, or to expect yourself to perform at this level without the counterbalance.

Add a new activity:

If you are over-focused on one activity, take some time to experiment with a new activity or skill to round out your

> "The great essentials of happiness are: something to do, something to love, and something to hope for."
> -Joseph Addison

AESOP=Adults Experiencing Special Operating Problems

> "Never turn down a new experience unless it's against the law or will get you in serious trouble."
>
> -*Life's Little Instruction Calendar, Vol 5*

interests. When AESOPs attempt to alter their patterns by dropping one activity abruptly without something to put in its place, they tend to create an uncomfortable vacuum, and the old activity will resurface to fill the void.

Reality check #1:

AESOPs can be like hamsters on a wheel, continually going faster and faster. Adults with SOP need to be willing to check in with loved ones to find out if they have been on one-track, tunnel vision paths to the exclusion of their families.

Reality check #2:

Have a mentor or coach, who is not afraid to lay it on the line, as the ultimate reality check. Ask this person to alert you if he or she sees you swinging out of balance.

Life purpose:

Chapter 28 • Balance In Life

AESOPs can benefit from investigating or reviewing their life purpose. This may lead to a spiritual strengthening, an assessment of talent, or a new awareness of how they could better use their time and energy. This type of contemplative activity by itself can allow balance to emerge.

Identify obsessions:

It is a short distance from the end of the continuum to falling off the continuum and being obsessed with something. If you find yourself totally fixated on running (or training for the triathlon, or rebuilding your website) to the exclusion of everything else in your life, you may have stepped completely off the continuum. At these times, you need to re-evaluate and re-balance yourself.

Keep the concept of balance in mind:

While it may be difficult to achieve the "normal" concept of balance in life, at least keep it in mind. A useful tool is the "PIES" chart. Visualize a pie cut into four pieces labeled: Physical, Intellectual, Emotional and Spiritual. List what you are doing for yourself to maintain balance in each of these areas. At the very least you should be able to recognize when one piece of your pie is skimpy or nonexistent and take steps to incorporate that piece back into your life.

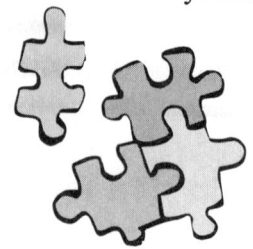

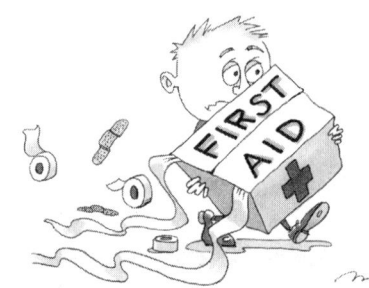

Need More First Aid?

If you can't balance your life because everything is piling up on top of you, see:
Chapter 1 on Overwhelm.

If you can't plan ahead, see:
Time Management in Chapter 5.

Chapter 28 • Balance In Life

If your life seems shallow and you feel you may need to add another dimension to it, see: **Chapter 34 on Spirituality.**

Wrapping It Up

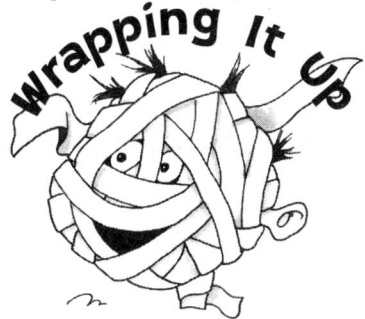

- For an AESOP, achieving balance in life requires an understanding of using extremes to create overall balance.

- AESOPs typically work hard for a period of time or focus intently on a project for a period of time. Their balance in life comes when they move away from the intense end of the continuum and allow time for decompression.

- This unique approach to life can be hard on the AESOP's partner and requires explanation and negotiation.

- It is imperative to watch out for extremes that move beyond the end of the continuum and into the range of obsessions or addictions.

AESOP=Adults Experiencing Special Operating Problems

Diet

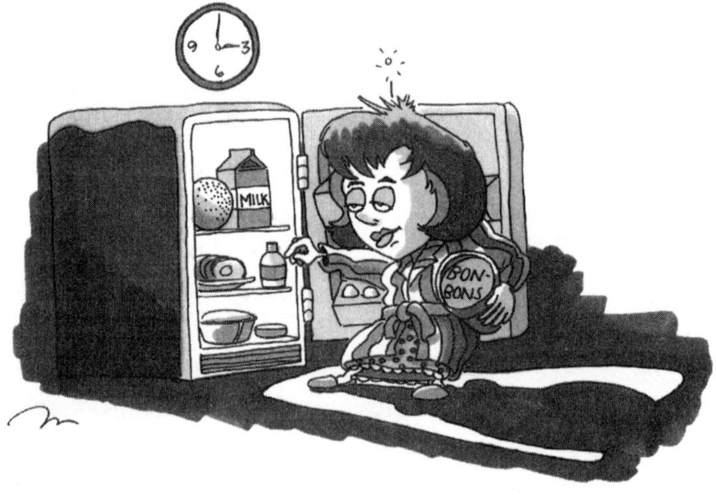

Chapter 29

What You Need To Know

Dieting is a major concern for most of the Western world; for AESOPs, it presents special challenges.

The AESOPs' biggest pitfalls with diet are:

- Filling each day to the brim, leaving no time to prepare meals or avoid fast food traps.
- Inconsistency: "Routine? What routine?"
- Night owl syndrome: late night grazing and sluggish mornings.
- All or nothing syndrome: yo-yoing between overdieting and overeating.

The Positive Spin

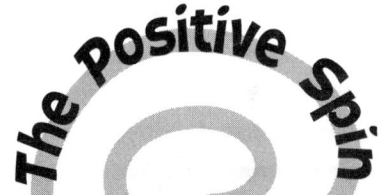

Drop the four letter word "diet" from your vocabulary. Instead, concentrate on changing your ideas about food. Approach health and weight by focusing on the way you buy food, the way you prepare food, and ideas to set yourself up for success. Accept the fact that, as AESOPs, we often do

 AESOP=Adults Experiencing Special Operating Problems

things in starts and stops. Mentally compliment yourself on what you do accomplish. If you totally fall apart and yield to the Del Taco drive-thru window at 10:00 PM , take a deep breath and start the process again.

> *"Come in, or we'll both starve." -Sign in a restaurant window*

Techniques

Pre-plan:

Stockpile nutritious, low calorie food in your home, office, and car. Buy in bulk and in quantities of more than one item so you won't run out. Consider breadsticks, pretzels, apples, low-fat cookies.

Embrace your inconsistency:

Since routines can be nearly impossible, use an energy burst to hardboil two dozen eggs, broil thirty-six chicken breasts, package twenty ready-to-go breakfasts. These will be available for times that all you can do is grab and run.

Practice Damage Control

When your AESOP nature

threatens to sabotage your healthy eating intentions, recognize the specific place in which problems are occurring.

Time damage control:

If your day is filled to the brim, it will be almost impossible to make even a quick stop to pick up fresh cottage cheese at the market. If your schedule is overloaded, you won't have the energy required to keep your personal health commitment. Be sure to allow extra time in your day for food emergencies and for meals, or well deserved nonfood down-time such as reading a good book or soaking in a bubble bath.

Depression damage control:

Watch out for those little things that can send you into a minor depression and steer clear! Weighing yourself constantly, comparing yourself to emaciated models, working out next to perfect bodies in leotards, or trying on bathing suits can completely overturn your resolve and bring on depression, making you feel hopeless. And feeling hopeless often brings on periods of overeating or bingeing. Protect yourself!

Grocery damage control:

Don't shop when you are hungry, and don't stock up on foods that will be tough to resist in the midnight hours. You won't be able to say no to yourself that frequently.

Night Owl damage control:

Many of us are midnight grazers. To combat that, force yourself to eat regularly and moderately throughout the day. This retrains your metabolism to expect food in small quantities rather than suppressing it all day and making up for it at night.

Environment damage control:

Set yourself up for success. Skip the morning breakfast meetings where jelly doughnuts and croissants are the only offerings. If you can't avoid the meeting, bring your own snack or bring a fruit plate for everyone; your example might start a trend! Reroute your drive home away from your favorite fast food stop or local yogurt shop.

yo-yo damage control:

Beware of diet plans that promise quick weight loss. Yes, crash diets often take off pounds quickly; unfortunately, these pounds return just as quickly. Much of the weight loss is water, or worse, muscle mass. Prepare yourself mentally for a long-term change in your habits rather than a short-term "diet." There is no quick fix in the world of food management.

Alaskan tundra damage control:

Our bodies are designed for survival. They are primitively hard-wired to store fat for long, hard winters and shed fat when food is more abundant. When we don't eat over a period of time, our bodies panic and begin to hold onto fat--for that long trek over the Alaskan tundra. This is where the complaint of "I'm hardly eating anything, and I'm still not losing

> "If chocolate could teach, I would by now be extremely well-educated."
>
> -Ashleigh Brilliant

weight" comes in. It's because we're hardly eating anything that our bodies hold on, instead of letting go. Balance, moderation, and consistency may be tough for AESOPs but they're still good long-range goals.

General damage control:

There will be days when controlling diet is the last thing on your mind. Know that if you give yourself permission to temporarily indulge, your "down-time" will be shorter. If this occurs, see it as an isolated period of time and don't doom the rest of the day. Remember the saying "what one resists, persists."

For Serious Weight Loss

If you have more than just a few pounds to shed, seek out a program that provides structure and support. Look for structure in the form of menus that are clear and can be incorporated into your own lifestyle. Look also for a program that provides a lecture once or twice a week where fellow

> "Never eat more than you can lift."
> -Miss Piggy

participants can get together and share stories. Knowing a support meeting is fast approaching (typically with a weigh-in) can be a powerful motivation. And don't forget about the food management secret weapon--exercise!

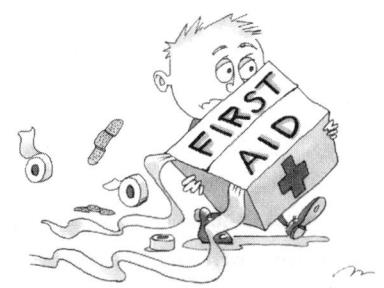

Need More First Aid?

If stress is a major factor in problems with diet, see: **Stress Reduction in Chapter 2.**

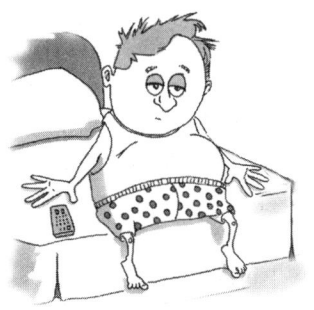

If you need more tools to change your lifestyle, see:

AESOP=Adults Experiencing Special Operating Problems

Balance in Life in Chapter 28.

If you need tips on incorporating exercise into your life, see:
Chapter 30 on Exercise.

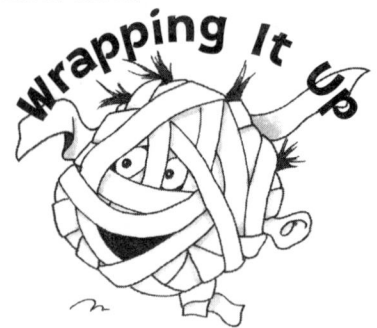

- Keeping healthy and maintaining a "good" weight for your own body type is an ongoing process.

- Adults with SOP need to consider their own particular routine, tendency to fill each day to the brim, and tendency toward depression.

- Techniques that include shopping strategies, preparing foods in quantity, and cutting down on midnight grazing will all help.

- Adults with SOP typically have trouble with consistency. Consider the starts and stops in any diet as part of your normal routine. When a stop occurs, pick yourself up, and start again with no recriminations.

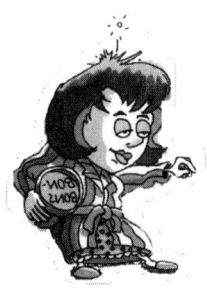

> "Be careful about reading health books. You may die of a misprint."
> -Mark Twain

Exercise

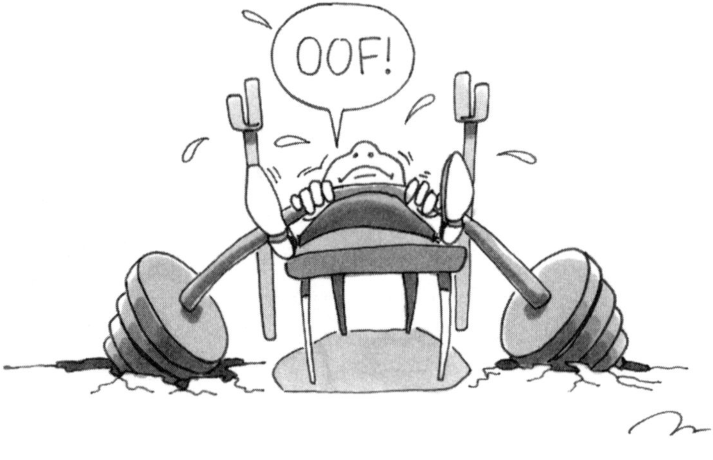

Chapter 30

What You Need To Know

Hooray for labor-saving devices in the modern world! These allow us to do just about anything without moving from our padded chairs. Unfortunately, our resulting inactivity can attract weight like a magnet and make exercise yet another extra something we have to plan for in our busy lives.

An AESOP's biggest pitfalls with exercise are:

- Filling each day to the brim, which leaves no time to exercise, right?
- Inconsistency: We get bored, we stop and start, we procrastinate.
- Night owl syndrome: "The only time I really feel like working out is 1:00 AM, but I can't work out at night, can I?"
- Early morning slug syndrome: "I should be able to work out at 5:30, right? Then why can't I get out of bed?"
- Lethargy or depression: "I feel so dragged down, I can't even get going."
- All-or-Nothing syndrome: We overdo it, which leads to injury which leads to no

AESOP=Adults Experiencing Special Operating Problems

workouts at all. Or if we don't have time for the 5-mile walk, we give up rather than taking the 1-mile walk.

● Menopause: This monumental phase of life makes exercise look like an impossibility.

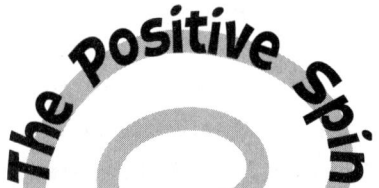

There are amazing benefits of regular exercise for AESOPs, not the least of which are changes in body chemistry and outlook.

Additionally, variety can be the spice of life in an AESOP's world. Having multiple options available can turn exercise from drudgery to play. Life holds creativity, pleasure, and fun; exercise gives you more years to enjoy them. And when the exercise itself holds variety, pleasure, and fun, you're getting double benefits!

Techniques
Pre-Plan:

A huge roadblock to exercising is the tendency to overfill the day and not keep open the time for exercise. We pay attention to so many tasks that our priorities can change by the minute and exercise often gets bumped to the last on the list. Remember, exercise is as important as getting enough sleep for feeling strong and confident in our lives, and therefore being able to do all those other tasks most effectively. So plan for your exercise, schedule it, and honor that time commitment!

Commit yourself:

Signing up for a class, having a personal trainer, or making a pact with a friend to work out serve as self-sabotage preventers that help us keep our promise to work out. When we've spent money or made a promise to a friend, we're more likely to follow through.

Embrace your inconsistency:

Stopping and starting exercise is an AESOP trait. We get bored! Keeping a routine is hard, and bad weather or

> "People treat their bodies as if they were rented."
> -Chungliang Al Huang

AESOP=Adults Experiencing Special Operating Problems

> "Success is not tomorrow; Success is today. Do it now! Get it done! Success is on the way."
> —*Life's Little Treasure Book On Hope*

broken equipment present tempting excuses for slacking off. The solution? Select two or three activities that you enjoy, so if one loses its appeal for awhile, there's an immediate back-up. As an example, you might belong to a gym, have a treadmill at home, and sign up for a class. This way you have multiple options available and fewer excuses to quit.

Recognize the Night Owl Syndrome:

Many AESOPs have unique body rhythms. "Experts" say we should exercise in the morning, but what if mornings are a nightmare for you? Rearrange your thinking about what you "should" be doing. Fitness and health don't care what time you exercise, they just respond to the fact that you are exercising. Many gyms have become 24-hour meccas for AESOP night owls; exercise equipment or videos in your home can happen at any hour. Honor your individual body rhythm.

Combat the early morning slug syndrome:

If waking up is painful and it occurs for you in layers, accept this as a part of your chemistry. Identify for yourself when you are the most alive and awake; this is the time an exercise program is most likely to work for you. Deciding to spend a half hour on the treadmill at 5:30 each morning when you can't even open your eyes is setting yourself up for failure.

Lethargy or depression damage control:

Many of us struggle with lethargy or depression that makes exercise look like an impossible mission. We fully understand that it would be good for us, that we'd feel a lot better, and that we'd benefit from the endorphins. The trouble is, we can't even get started. One possible solution is focusing on the memory of how exercise has made you feel better in the past. Then concentrate on how to replicate that feeling. Or you might consider laying out your sweatshirt, pants, socks, and shoes in a trail leading away from your bed or couch and toward the front door. When the alarm rings, you're ready to go!

Congratulate yourself for every effort:

Walk out the door and around the block, and then reward yourself for getting it done. Building on even this small success encourages future walks and gets a routine going. You don't have to get elaborate; just get out the door. By the way, having an event to look forward to can be a wonderful motivator. An upcoming dance, hike, or cruise can be great reasons to get fit; so can participating in sponsored walks for your favorite charity, such as leukemia or breast-cancer research.

All-or-nothing damage control:

Ever plunge headlong into an exercise program, working out several hours a day or week, only to pull a muscle and be laid up with an injury for a month that prohibits all exercise? One thing AESOPs can be is driven, and being driven to exercise can be a problem. When we overdo exercise and injure ourselves, we'll be forced to quit until our muscles recover. So patience, patience, patience! Start slowly and build. We're talking about long-term successful exercise, not the yo-yo effect between driving yourself too hard and then cooling your heels over an ice pack.

Menopause damage control:

It is unbelievable how many women still don't get the importance and impact of menopause. Unfortunately, this is reinforced by a medical community and a societal view that doesn't teach about the impact that menopause has in a woman's life. In

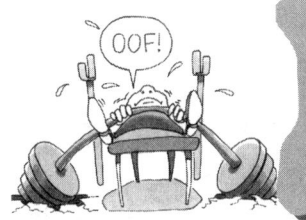

"The only reason I would take up jogging is so that I could hear heavy breathing again." *-Erma Bombeck*

menopause, the chemistry of the body changes and the metabolism slows even more (if that's possible). Depression and lethargy rear their ugly heads even more frequently. The level of estrogen in the body changes. Muscles that used to bounce back quickly now ache with exercise. Knees crack when you stand up.

The first thing to do is pick up a good book on menopause for some information and a positive perspective. Recognize that if twenty minutes of exercise three times a week were enough to keep you in a size twelve dress at age twenty-five, it will take forty minutes of exercise five times a week in your fifties to do the same thing. Fight the tendency to stop exercising at menopause if you have an exercise program in place. If you don't exercise

> "Observe your dog: if he's fat, you're not getting enough exercise."
>
> -*Quips & Quotes*

Chapter 30 • Exercise

yet, start with a lighter impact program. You can always work up from there.

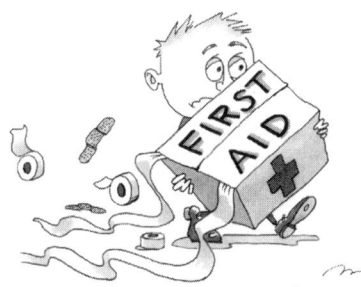

Need More First Aid?

If managing your time (or lack of it) plays a big part in not exercising, see:
Time Management in Chapter 5.

If you just don't seem to get around to exercising, see:
Procrastination in Chapter 6.

If you want more information on how or why exercise is important, see:
Balance in Life in Chapter 28.

If you are female and your exercise habits and body chemistry have changed over the years, see:
Menopause in

Chapter 36. Wrapping It Up

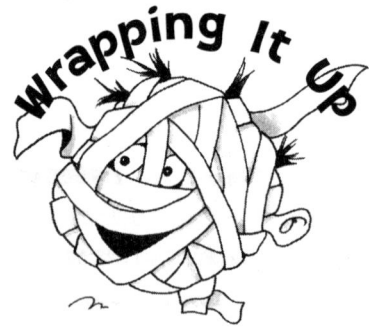

- As AESOPs, we have certain pitfalls to exercising such as filling each day to the brim, stopping and starting routines, having touchy body chemistries, and having an all-or-nothing philosophy.

- Variation in types of exercise is essential to combat the boredom and increase the fun.

- There are techniques and tips available to tackle your particular exercise pitfalls.

- Even though we live in a labor-saving-device world, exercise remains a critical part of a healthy mind and body.

> "Life holds creativity, pleasure, and fun; exercise gives you more years to enjoy them. And when the exercise itself holds variety, pleasure, and fun, you're getting double benefits!"
>
> *-Joan and Denise*

AESOP=Adults Experiencing Special Operating Problems

Sleep

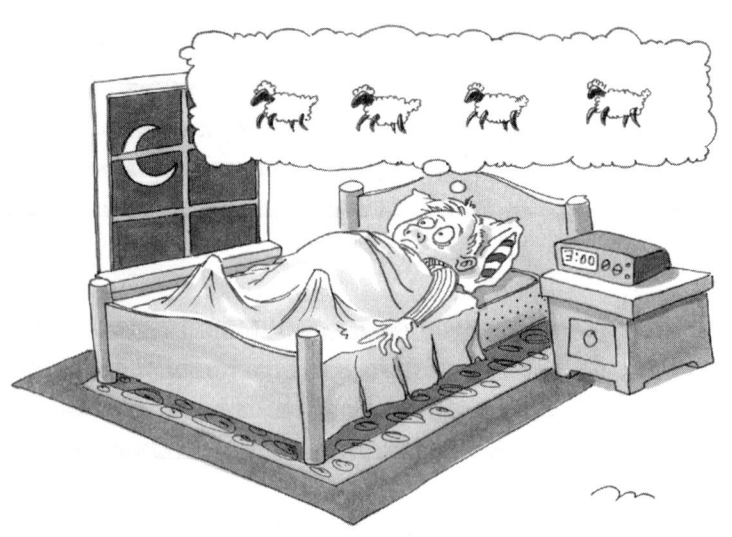

Chapter 31

What You Need To Know

Sleep problems can be a common complaint among AESOPs. Sleep problems show up most often in three ways:

- Can't get to sleep. 1 AM, 2 AM, 3 AM, here I am watching the clock again. Can't I ever go to sleep?
- Don't want to go to sleep! There's something magical and compelling about the night. It may be a sense of finally being alone, a sense of adventure, of being out on the fringe of dark, feeling a "pull" from the night and never wanting it to end.
- Sleep seems like such a waste of time! We may resist sleep because finally falling asleep sets us up to face another chaotic day.
- Once asleep, we're dead to the world and can't wake up. It's that feeling of sinking into a million feather beds. Once out, we're gone for the duration, not even waking up for earthquakes, fire alarms, and certainly not for alarm clocks. (In contrast, a small percentage of Adults with SOP sleep

AESOP=Adults Experiencing Special Operating Problems

so lightly that even snails tracking across a window pane wake them up.)

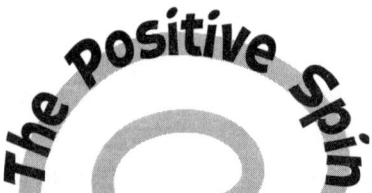

The Positive Spin

We may have horrible memories of being a kid lying in bed looking at the ceiling for hours because our parents wanted us in bed at a "decent hour," and then told us it was our fault that we couldn't get up for school in the morning. As Adults with SOP, we need to accept that our sleep patterns may be the result of a genetic predisposition that needs to be respected and dealt with. Notice that many of the tools in this section aren't about fixing us, but rather are about working with our sleeping patterns.

Techniques
Tools to Get to Sleep

Sleep devices:

Sometimes sound and/or motion machines work, based on our individual preferences. Consider these: lava lamps, white noise machines, circulating fans, playing certain music, setting the TV on a timer.

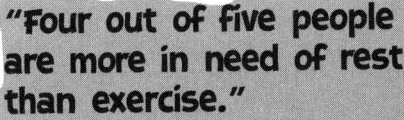

> "Four out of five people are more in need of rest than exercise."
> -Dr. Logan Clendening

Foods/Herbs:

Warm milk, turkey (with its sleep inducing tryptophan), decaffeinated or herbal tea, sleep aids found at the local health food store may work. If all else fails we may need prescribed medication to sleep. If so, we need to consult our physician.

Winding down:

Try getting into a warm bath or hot tub, learning self-hypnosis, or using relaxation or meditation tapes. Remember to allow time for sleep to happen. Expecting to go to sleep in five or ten minutes when sleep has been a problem isn't realistic.

Tools for the Night Owl

Communicate:

We need to use our best

communication skills to explain our sleep patterns so that our significant other doesn't feel rejected when we don't go to bed at the same time.

Be considerate:

We need to be aware that rattling around at night (watching TV, slamming a cupboard door) may keep our roommates or partners up, which will cause problems in our relationships.

Examine work schedules:

We need to explore whether a graveyard or swing shift is available in our jobs, and whether a change would better match our bodies' rhythms to our working/sleeping cycles.

Nap often:

We can use catnaps during the day to provide renewed energy and make up for the sleep deprivation night owls often experience. Naps should generally take place before late afternoon to avoid triggering your nighttime sleep cycle. Usually thirty to sixty minutes is more than enough.

Be conscious of your peak productivity hours and capitalize on them:

As we work with our sleep

> "Remember that almost everything looks better after a good night's sleep."
> -*Life's Little Treasure Book On Hope*

patterns, we will still need to produce a certain amount of work at home or on the job. We need to become aware of our peak productivity times of day, afternoon or evening, and reserve those times in our schedule for high-priority tasks.

Tools for Waking Up

Alarm clocks:

We need to test our sensitivity to certain alarm clocks before we buy. One method to consider: buy alarm clocks of varying pitch and intensity that you *do* react to. Set these clocks at increasing distances from the bed, so that you have to take physical steps to turn them off.

Research different types of alarms:

There are alarms that shriek, whistle, or increase in volume each time we hit the snooze button. There are

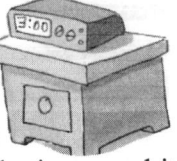

> "The last time I felt good was at 10:00 AM about nine years ago."
> -Ashleigh Brilliant

alarms that we can place under our pillow or bedding that vibrate us awake. There are alarms that simulate increasing brightness to mimic the sun. Check them out!

Partner or spouse as alarm:

If we count on our partners to wake us up, we need to remember an important rule: we are not allowed to get mad at them for waking us up! They are doing what we requested and don't deserve our crankiness. This method of waking up must be carefully negotiated and mutually agreed upon, or it will cause more problems than it is worth.

Wake-up service:

There are companies that specialize in helping us wake up. They operate like hotels, calling to alert us to the time. They can be instructed to call more than once!

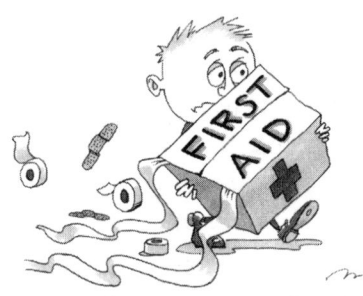

Need More First Aid?

If you still have trouble with lateness as it relates to sleep, see:
Late Again in Chapter 14.

If your sleeping patterns are causing trouble in your relationship, see:
Help for Yourself and/or Help for Your Partner and Family in Chapters 21 and 22.

If your sleeping pattern differences affect your sex life, see:
Sex in Chapter 24.

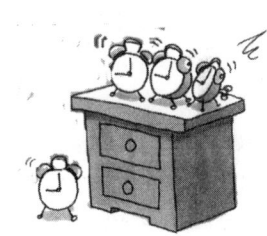

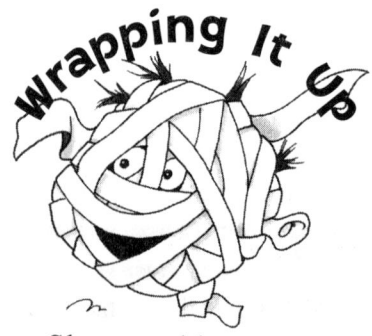

Wrapping It Up

- Sleep problems are a common complaint among AESOPs.

- The usual problems are not being able to get to sleep, not wanting to go to sleep, or not being able to wake up once we get to sleep.

- We can experiment with sleep devices, foods/herbs, and winding down to help us get to sleep.

- There are special considerations for the night owl.

- Various alarm clocks and tools such as wake-up services can help us at the other end of sleep.

- There is hope for us if our sleep patterns have been a problem--we are not alone!

Chapter 31 • Sleep

> "As Adults with SOP, we need to accept that our sleep patterns may be the result of a genetic predisposition that needs to be respected and dealt with."
>
> *-Joan and Denise*

AESOP=Adults Experiencing Special Operating Problems

Hyperactivity vs. Hypoactivity

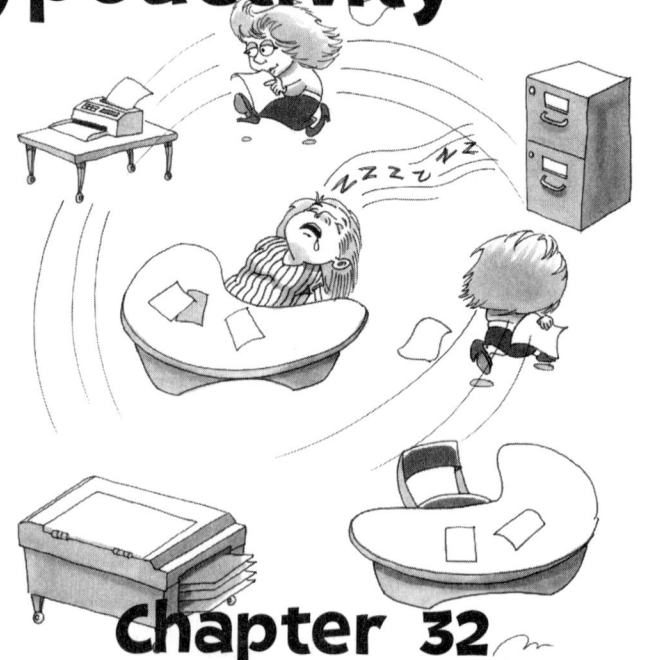

chapter 32

What You Need To Know

Your typical speed is faster than lightening, and the rest of the world seems to be in slow motion. People can't understand why you never hold still, and you can't understand why they don't hurry up! You may not even know how to explain that there's a motor running inside of you. You are hyperactive.

On the other side of the coin, you are in SLOW motion as the world whips by. People don't understand why it takes you so long to get your thoughts together, to get them out, or just to get moving! Your intentions are good, you just can't seem to kick into gear. You are hypoactive.

Even more confusing, not only to yourself but also to other people, you may be a combination of both. It is not uncommon to hear people talk about being filled with energy upon awakening, only to find themselves with the energy of a deflated balloon by noon. You may experience surges of hyperactivity alternating with

AESOP=Adults Experiencing Special Operating Problems

hypoactivity; one of the most frustrating aspects is how unpredictable these cycles are.

The Positive Spin

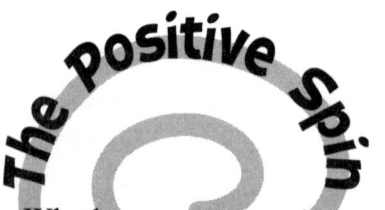

Whether you experience hyperactivity, hypoactivity or a combination of both, you are struggling with biochemistry. Your body is unique, and what might work for you may not work for another person. We can't really expect non-AESOP adults to understand hyperactivity or hypoactivity; they just don't know what it feels like inside our bodies. What we can do is appreciate our own body chemistries (even if no one else seems to!) and work with them instead of against them. With specific coping skills we can shift or adapt some aspects of our body chemistry and its consequences without losing track of who we truly are at the core.

Techniques
Overall Body Care to Balance our Chemistry

> "There is more to life than increasing its speed." -*Mahatma Gandhi*

Consider rest:

Often, just taking a breather from our routines can clear our minds and change our body cycles. A quick nap, closing our eyes for a minute to block out stimuli, or putting our feet up can reset our body rhythms.

Look at nutrition that supports your biochemistry:

Buy a cooler. Get pre-packaged meals that are healthy. Make up foods and freeze them for later in the week. Know where the salad bars are at fast food restaurants in town. Carefully monitoring and then attending to your nutritional needs can directly influence your energy and therefore your activity levels.

Get regular medical check ups:

Don't leave your doctor's office without setting up your next appointment or filling out a reminder card. If you don't take care of your next visit while the opportunity is in front of you, it will be "out of sight, out of mind," and your medication or health visits may lapse.

Exercise:

Exercise changes the biochemistry of the brain. Rather than waiting to set up an elaborate work-out plan, remember that any motion at all is better than none. So park at the far end of the mall and walk. Do ten sit-ups. Choose the stairs. If you decide to launch into a full exercise regimen, be prepared to stop and start again frequently. Your commitment is to come back to exercise.

Many of the following activities are traditionally done at either high-intensity or low-intensity. For the hyperactive person, these activities may calm you down; for the hypoactive person, they may energize you. Don't hesitate to try them,

> "If a man watches more than three football games in a row, he should be declared legally dead."
> -Erma Bombeck

and stick with what works. You may even find yourself enjoying it!

- *High-intensity activities*: Power-walking, cycling, jogging, using a Nordic Track, dancing, race car or go-cart driving, swimming, or any physical work-out so intense that it leaves you winded and tired when finished; physical labor such as painting a room, wall papering, shoveling, pruning trees; amusement park roller coaster/thrill rides, that leave you breathless with your heart pounding.

- *Low-intensity activities*: Journal writing; quiet hobbies such as crossword puzzles or needlepoint; seeing a pleasant movie; practicing meditation or prayer; napping; taking a hot shower or a dip in a Jacuzzi; reading or listening to soothing music.

Accepting Our Chemistry

Work on self-acceptance:

Although advances in health and science are moving rapidly,

the best thing we can do for ourselves in adjusting to our body chemistry is to practice accepting ourselves for who and how we are. Begin by identifying your unique body state(s). Next, learn to recognize when your unique chemistry may be affecting how you operate in your world. Third, begin an acceptance/compromise dialogue with yourself. For example, you might say, "OK, today I feel so hypoactive, I don't want

> "Do what you can with what you have, where you are."
> -Theodore Roosevelt

to get going. I'll make a deal with myself to make two phone calls so at the end of the day I still feel like I've accomplished something. Tomorrow will be a better day."

Recognize that self-berating is harmful:

We often spend time kicking ourselves for who and how we are. Realize that being mean and

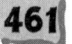

judgmental with yourself not only stops productive action, it may even worsen your biochemistry.

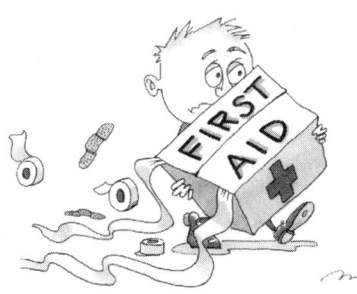

Need More First Aid?

If your physical state leaves you feeling blue a lot of the time, see:
Moods in Chapter 16 and Depression in Chapter 17.

If you need more tips on how to balance your body, see:
Stress Reduction in Chapter 2 and Balance in Life in Chapter 28.

If you need specific tips to deal with common problem areas for the hyperactivity and/or hypoactivity, see:
Diet in Chapter 29, Exercise in Chapter 30,

and Sleep in Chapter 31.

If you need help calming and centering yourself, see: **Spirituality in Chapter 34.**

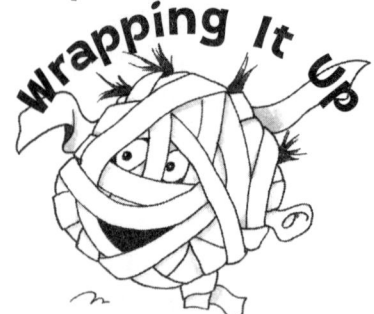

- Hyperactivity and hypoactivity can be opposite ends of the AESOP continuum.

- We may also have a combination of both, which may be confusing and require special coping skills.

- Both hyperactivity and hypoactivity are a result of biochemistry.

- There are a variety of areas that affect our biochemistry and can help balance it out, including rest, nutrition, keeping on top of our medical check-ups, and exercise, both high-intensity and low-intensity.

- AESOPs often berate ourselves for who and how we are. It's important to stop making matters worse by condemning the way we were made.

- Self-acceptance and coping skills go a long way in successfully dealing with hyperactivity and hypoactivity.

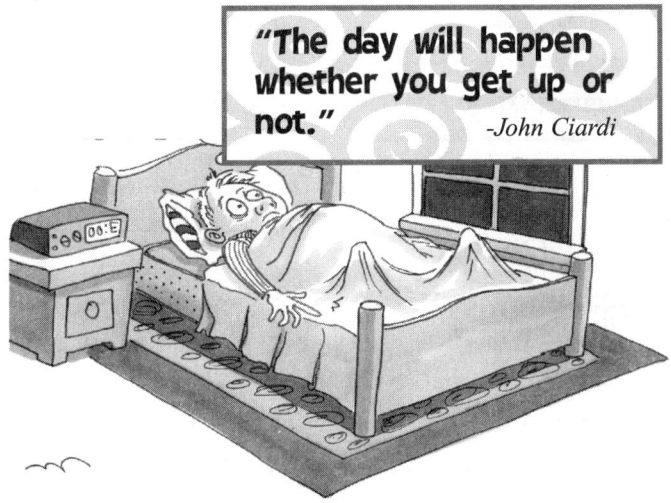

"The day will happen whether you get up or not."
-*John Ciardi*

AESOP=Adults Experiencing Special Operating Problems

Addictions

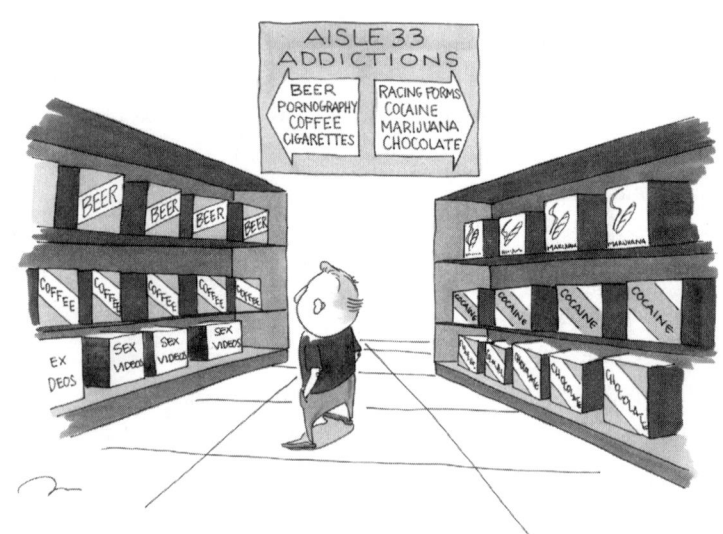

Chapter 33

What You Need To Know

Addictions are a major concern for AESOPs. The Adult with SOP is constantly fighting a bio-chemical imbalance. Our systems just don't feel right; instead, we seem somehow off-kilter. In fact, from day to day we may be aware of a variation in our ability to think or perform. If we happen to encounter something, anything at all, that stabilizes our systems, understandably, we want to return again and again to that "normal" feeling. We may find that three cups of coffee in the morning help us to get to work on time and organize our day. We may find that the small amount of Dexedrine found in a common prescription diet pill seems to clear the fuzziness from our brains. We may move on to more serious drugs and discover that a drug like marijuana allows us to calm down and appear normal (at least on the outside) for the first time in our lives. The trouble occurs as the Adults with SOP begin to use more and more of these

AESOP=Adults Experiencing Special Operating Problems

substances. Three cups of coffee doesn't set off any alarms, but when the coffee increases to three pots a day, there is a potential for physical harm. Two or three months' use of diet pills may not be alarming, but when AESOPs find themselves going from doctor to doctor to ensure a steady supply of "diet pills," there is a problem, particularly because of the added onset of shame and guilt. When a glass of wine with dinner becomes a bottle of wine to relax and unwind, we'd better start looking at the potential for addiction. Marijuana and other street drugs carry their own set of risks. They are not regulated in any way and can be considered a form of Russian roulette. Also, their potential for addiction is very real. As Wendy Richardson's <u>The Link Between ADD and Addictions</u> reminds us,""No one knows exactly how much heat, fuel, and wind it takes to

> **"The chains of habit are too weak to be felt until they are too strong to be broken."**
> -*Samuel Johnson*

Chapter 33 • Addictions

turn a burning cigarette into a forest fire."

AESOPs may also be severely at risk for addiction because of genetic markers present in our own DNA. As we understand more and more about genetics, we realize that if an individual carries one or more of the genes for addictions, even very limited use of a substance can propel us into full-blown addiction. Current research indicates that the genes present in many Adults with SOP and the genes for addiction are closely related.

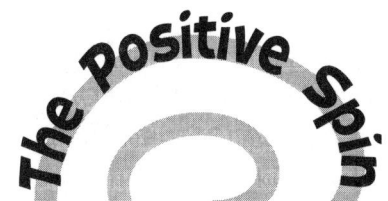

The Positive Spin

Our goal here is to shift the views on addiction from the helplessness to the courage to search for successful treatment.

In this day and age, addictions are understood to be "diseases" or "illnesses." While this is certainly an advancement from previous generations' condemnation of addictions as a moral flaw, it does not accurately portray the special set of circumstances and challenges present for the AESOP. In fact, the traditional concept of addictions being diseases or illnesses is an oversimplification for the AESOP population. AESOPs have an extremely difficult task as we constantly seek out substances (from benign to lethal) in our attempt to balance a difficult body chemistry. We must understand this constant flirting with addiction as a biochemical problem. If we don't recognize this, we can easily fall into the shadows of shame and guilt. Shame and guilt in turn can cause the AESOP to go underground rather than face our unique body chemistry head-on and courageously search for the treatment that will safely stabilize us and allow us success in life.

Techniques
Addressing the Question of Medication
Medication--Yes or No?

You must take a hard look at whether or not you will seek professional help including medication to deal with your biochemical imbalance. If your system is just a little out of whack, you may be able to get by without medication. If your imbalance is severe, the possibility of medication should be included in your treatment plan and may include one or more medications.

If you've flirted with addictions:

If your body chemistry is enough out of whack that you find yourself constantly moving from one substance to another in the hopes of finding something that brings you balance, you are flirting with addiction. Be mindful; this constant searching may signal that proper medication might be a safer or more reliable option for stabilizing your system.

If you know you've been addicted:

If you have been addicted, you may fear that taking any kind of medication will give you the same sort of edgy or stoned feeling that you had while using, and may even throw you back into addiction. Current research assures us that many previously addicted

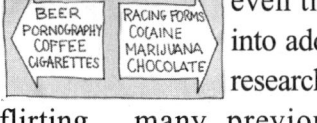

AESOPs can be successfully treated with proper medication. Other AESOPs who have struggled with addiction simply cannot tolerate certain medications, as they cause reactions too similar to the addiction itself and place us at risk for relapse. Careful monitoring by the AESOP, a physician, and a therapist who understands the link between SOP and addictions helps to provide a safety net for those of us who can include the use of medication in our treatment plan.

Be aware of the current 12-Step philosophy:

Traditionally, 12-Step programs have been opposed to the use of any medication (especially stimulants) as a potential threat to the recovery process. Within the last 10 years, 12-Step philosophy has slowly changed to recognize that a chemical imbalance is often present and medication may be needed to ensure continued progress in recovery.

> "Suffering isn't ennobling, recovery is."
> *-Christian Barnard*

With or Without Medication

Addictions take many different forms. Consider using the following categories as a guide:

Category I--Positive Addictions

Examples: exercise, meditation, yoga

Category I addictions are not generally considered harmful.

Dealing with Category I addictions

- Consider Plan A: Many AESOPs very successfully regulate their body chemistries with activities such as running or yoga.

However, there is danger here if family and work are shoved to one side, if the body is pushed beyond its limits, or if there is no back up plan in place when injuries or problems occur.

- Have a Plan B in place: This might include alternate forms of exercise, or negotiating with your family to include them in your exercise plan.

- Consider Plan C as well: Have an arrangement with your spouse or workout buddy to let you know when you are pushing the limit with either time or body strain so that you can back off before you crash.

Category II--Non Life-Threatening Addictions

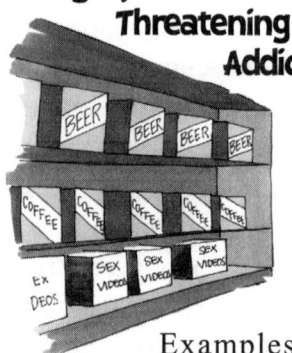

Examples: coffee, tea, espresso, Coca Cola, Mountain Dew, Excedrin

Category II includes substances Adults with SOP have happened upon in life that seem to provide energy, clear out the cobwebs and make the quality of life appear better. Many of these substances are not harmful in themselves and certainly not when used in moderation. However, "moderation" is not a word in most AESOPs' vocabularies, and excessive use of Category II substances can lead to real physical problems.

Dealing with Category II addictions

●Monitor your habits: If your need for a substance is constantly increasing (for example, if your Pepsi intake has jumped to a six-pack a day) consider switching to a different, more positive addiction such as exercise to regulate body chemistry. Also consider the use of medication.

- Be aware of *self*-medicating: People often self-medicate for years with coffee, coke or Excedrin, thinking that it is doing the job of stimulating and focusing them. In reality, prescription medication is far more effective and less harmful to the system. Using caffeine to medicate an AESOP is the equivalent of using a sledgehammer to crack a walnut instead of a nutcracker which would be more appropriate.

- Drink more water: Try drinking more water to flush out your liver and kidneys. The substances mentioned in Category II can be hard on your filtration system, and your body can always use more water.

- Look around for the "triggers" in your day: What situations cause enough stress to make you want these things? Is it getting up in the morning? An afternoon slump? Too many phone calls? Dealing with the reason that is behind the need can reduce that need.

Category III--Dangerous Addictions (Life-Threatening over Time)

Examples: diet pills, cigarettes, Percodan, Xanax, Alcohol

Category III examples may be viewed as extensions of Category II substances because they also produce a perceived positive effect in the body chemistry. Once again, AESOPs, may have happened upon these substances by chance. For example, a cigarette may surprisingly produce an extremely calming effect. Percodan, originally prescribed for pain, may increase the ability to focus and clear up the "fuzzy-headed" feeling. The innocently found results of these substances may lead to excessive use and ultimately abuse.

Dealing with Category III addictions

- Check your genes: If there is a family history of addiction, even short term use of a substance like Vicodin to relieve the pain of a back injury can set you up for addiction in short order. Check with your doctor for a safer substitute.

- **Watch your response:** You may find that Vicodin or Percodan make you feel extremely clear-headed and able to function. If so, this may be a signal that your unique SOP will respond positively to medical treatment, which should be pursued.

- **Risk honesty:** If you have used diet pills to consciously manage your SOP rather than to regulate your weight, be aware that many times these do work marginally. However, the shame and guilt over "misusing" a drug may often leave you feeling like an addict when in fact you have been self-medicating. Once you become aware of this, you can consult with your doctor for a medication that will more effectively and directly treat your SOP.

- **Be vigilant:** If you find yourself increasing your use of alcohol or cigarettes or if you are increasing the amount of your pain-killing medication "to get it to

AESOP=Adults Experiencing Special Operating Problems

work better," be mindful that these are danger signs. The SOP body chemistry may need to be properly medicated. If it is not, the tendency to increase use of harmful addictive substances will increase.

Category IV - Dangerous Addictions (Life-Threatening)

Examples: Cocaine, Speed, Crack, Ecstasy, Heroin.

The substances in this category are readily available out on the street in quantity, carry legal consequences, and have chemical make-ups which are uncertain and unregulated.

Dealing With Category IV addictions

● Move away from shame and guilt: It cannot be emphasized enough, most AESOPs have biochemical imbalances in the brain, not weaknesses in character. Realize that Adults with SOP, particularly if a genetic trigger is present, can have a high drive to self-medicate.

● What to do about your substance use/abuse: The first step is acknowledging that you have a problem of over-using a substance. You will be starting a journey that may include

> "God gave us the grace to accept with serenity the things that cannot be changed; courage to change the things that should be changed; and the wisdom to distinguish the one from the other."
>
> —*Reinhold Niebuhr*

reading, getting professional help, attending 12-Step programs, and possibly medication. For many AESOPs medication is a necessary aspect of treatment. With proper medication, your tendency to self-medicate may begin to subside. Be prepared that your physician may change or moderate your prescriptions to find the most effective dose. This does not indicate that you are unusually difficult or beyond hope, so don't feel you should therefore revert to your former substances. Get support to keep all aspects of your treatment plan in focus.

- Who to go to when you are in trouble: Start with a trusted ally who recognizes your request for help as a call for supportive referrals to appropriate diagnosticians in your area. When consulting your physician, ask that your tendency towards addiction be taken into consideration when medication is discussed. If you don't have a physician, pre-screen to locate one with expertise in addictions as well as your particular SOP. If you have addiction in your background, you will most likely need the services of a psychiatrist.

- What to expect: Even with a diagnosis, physicians are often reluctant to prescribe any medication, especially a stimulant, to someone with a history or a tendency towards addiction. Many physicians will start with low doses of an anti-depressant, gradually increasing the dose. They may also advice or even insist on counseling and 12-Step program participation as adjunct therapies.

- Consult SOP-knowledgeable attorneys: If you are in trouble with the law because of drugs, sometimes an official written diagnosis can shift the way your case is viewed by the court. This is especially true if you are seeking treatment.

- Relapse is a major concern for people in recovery: Recognize that clean and sober AESOPs may feel on the verge of impending relapse when AESOP traits are acting up. Depression, fuzzy thinking, lack of motivation and social isolation may not be signs of relapse at all, just signals that our chemistry is out of balance. Unfortunately, people in the recovery field don't always recognize this phenomenon.

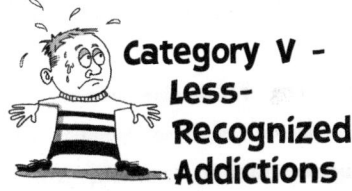

Category V - Less-Recognized Addictions

Examples: Sexual addiction, Anorexia, Bulimia, compulsive overeating, gambling, thrill-seeking, electronic addictions to the Internet or email.

Even though the addictions in this category may appear separate and distinct on the surface, they have some commonalties. The techniques listed below can be used as general guidelines:

Dealing with Category V addictions:

- Acknowledge your tendencies: Often only you can monitor when something moves from occasional to habitual or addictive use. However, be open to feedback from family and friends who will often comment on losing your time or attention to the addiction.

- Read up on your addiction: Reading various kinds of information on your particular addiction can help you further define the extent of the problem and open doors to possible resources.

- Explore your family history: Addictions frequently are linked to genetics. Look at behaviors and patterns within the family system. This can often help you confirm your own suspicion that you have an addiction and also reinforce the message that you are not alone.

- Consider professional help: Be aware that there are physicians, therapists, groups, and even hospitals that specialize in addiction rehabilitation.

- Consider the role of medication: If you are an AESOP, diagnosed or not, who is self-medicating with addictive substances or behaviors, the use of properly prescribed medication may be extremely helpful. Be open to including medication in your treatment.

- Locate a 12-Step meeting in your area: Receiving support from fellow recovering people who share your addictive behavior can feel like being in an accepting family. 12-Step programs also offer a semi-structured format to help you come to grips and cope with your addiction.

- A special word about sexual addictions: Where do you draw the line between healthy sexuality and sexual addiction? We are bombarded with sexual images in the media, which tend to confuse the issue. What is normal and what is too much when it comes to sexual thoughts? Dr. Patrick Carnes lists the SAFE formula for telling when thoughts of sex could move into the realm of a sexual addiction:

AESOP=Adults Experiencing Special Operating Problems

Secret--Is your behavior secret?

Abusive--Is it abusive to self or others?

Feelings--Are your feelings too painful, or do you avoid them through sexual acting out?

Empty--Do you feel empty or devoid of a caring loving relationship?

Sexual addiction is an area where support in terms of a 12-Step group and professional counseling as well as help for your partner is a must.

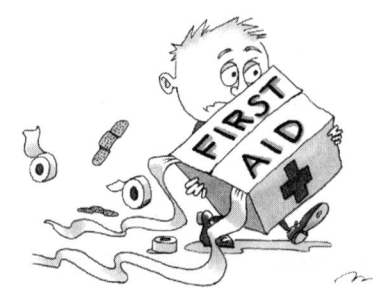

Need More First Aid?

If you impulsively reach for substances or turn to harmful behaviors to make you feel better, see:

Impulsivity in Chapter 9.

If you're just not sure how your life is supposed to work

Chapter 33 • Addictions

smoothly, see:
Balance in Life in Chapter 28.

If you need ideas for exercise as a more positive addiction alternative, see:
Exercise in Chapter 30.

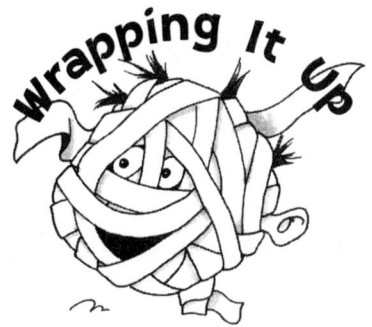

- AESOPs are often vulnerable to addictive substances or behaviors.

- Substance use is often an attempt to self-medicate body chemistry that's out of whack.

- The use of prescribed medication should be carefully considered.

- There are different categories of addictions ranging from relatively harmless to life threatening.

- Addictions can include such things as gambling, eating

AESOP=Adults Experiencing Special Operating Problems

disorders, sex, and electronic games.

- Educating yourself, using qualified professional help, and considering 12-Step support programs can all provide a solid recovery base.

> "AESOPs have an extremely difficult task as we constantly seek out substances (from benign to lethal) in our attempt to balance a difficult body chemistry. We must understand this constant flirting with addiction as a biochemical problem."
>
> *-Joan and Denise*

AESOP=Adults Experiencing Special Operating Problems

Spirituality

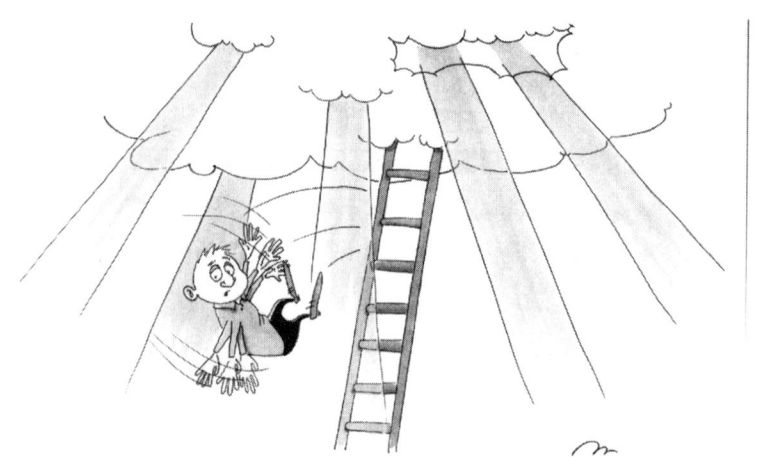

Chapter 34

What You Need To Know

AESOPs often have unique belief systems, sometimes far from those of mainstream society. This may include our belief systems about spirituality.

The term "spirituality" is often associated with a traditional church or religion. You may or may not have had a positive experience with organized religion as a child. Churches and temples are often made up of many Adults without SOP.

Sometimes SOP children are placed in rigid and demanding environments. As adults, they may recall voices from the past telling them to "Sit still. Listen. Follow along. Get along with others. Don't tap your feet." Because they couldn't conform, they may have felt a sense of disapproval or felt that they were bad or lacking spirituality.

Often Adults with SOP value their alone time or may be loners. For them, the thought of sitting trapped in a church for an hour surrounded by people while attempting to listen to a

AESOP=Adults Experiencing Special Operating Problems

sermon (with all kinds of thoughts racing through their heads) is something to avoid.

If this is true for you, you may choose to develop your own unique brand of spirituality. However, if you are comfortable in a traditional church or religious setting, lean into and strengthen your faith, accepting your SOP as yet another part of you. Your church home may serve as an important social outlet where you can come together with others of your faith and be supported through life's trials and tribulations.

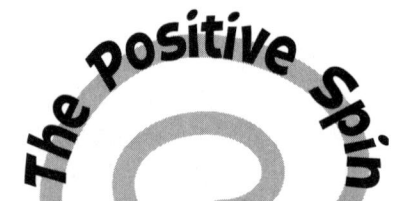

There can be a much broader definition of the word "spirit" than what is used by many religions. Spirit can be seen as a vital or animated source, or as the soul. The idea of spirit can bring to mind the inter-connectedness of all things. As humans, we can trace the need for spirituality back to our earliest times. This suggests that spirituality is a necessary part of the human

> "If you want to remain in touch with the spiritual side of life, you have to be flexible enough to follow the direction of the journey as the journey itself changes direction."
> -*Phil Catalfo*

condition for health, both physically and mentally.

AESOPs are unique and creative in their thought processes. Their creativity enables them to see things from a different perspective, or to come up with a brand new idea. AESOPs who find a traditional church or temple too confining may need to step outside of the conventional and search elsewhere for their answers. Again, if your faith has sustained you all your life, embrace it fully. But, if you're still searching, don't give up.

Be creative in seeking out your own sources of spirituality. Look for what is right for you, not just what is traditional or commonly accepted. Are you more at peace and in touch with your Higher Power when you are alone? Are you the type of person who needs the support of other adults who care about you? Recognize your own uniqueness as an AESOP. Don't be afraid to seek out your very own unique solution to fulfill the need for spirituality.

Adults with SOP are often faced with challenges in life, and at times it seems impossible to gather the strength to keep on plugging away at life, to continue moving forward. Often spiritual strength provides the resources we need. For the AESOP, it must be a spirituality that fits with our own belief system. It must be a spirituality that fits with our own need for peace and grounding in life. Remember, spirituality can be found in music, chants, nature, meditation, prayer, and sacred dance as well as in formal serv-

> "Here is the test to find whether your mission on earth is finished. If you're alive, it isn't."
> -Richard Bach

ices. Keep your spirit open to possibilities that will allow you extra strength.

Techniques
Tools for the Traditionally Minded

Find a church that fits:

Are you typically late? Do you move and shift around if you have to sit in one place for longer than 15 minutes? Find a church or temple that fits your brand of SOP.

Persist until you feel accepted:

Look for an environment where you are accepted just as you are, with all your flaws. Look for an organization or congregation that is non-judgmental and accepting. If you have any negative feelings in the pit of your stomach while attending a particular church, it isn't the place for you.

Embrace your uniqueness:

The rest of the world may believe one way. Yet, because of the inner twists and turns your mind takes, you may choose to develop your own unique style of spirituality and worship. Realize that

> "I know God will not give me anything I can't handle. I just wish that He didn't trust me so much."
> -Mother Teresa

this is just fine.

Embrace the pain in growth:

People with SOP are exceptionally creative, and frequently challenge their lives, their relationships, and their belief systems. See this challenge as a normal function for you. It doesn't matter that you have believed X, Y, or Z for the last twenty-five years. You may have progressed to a different level of awareness, and you may need to re-examine your spirituality. See this as a positive challenge rather than questioning whether there is something wrong with you.

Dealing with family:

Your family may not understand your drives to explore your spirituality. Assess whether your family is accepting and open-minded enough to understand your spiritual position and respect it as your own, even if they believe differently. If you have this type of family, you are lucky. On the other hand, if telling your family about your beliefs will be an uphill battle, decide if the outcome is worth the journey. If your family is such that hurt feelings, anger, and even outrage will appear, take that into consideration. At times it is enough to know inside that you are comfortable and at peace.

Beware of "Good, God-fearing, church-going people":

Some (certainly not all) people who profess to be spiritual hold themselves up as having a special set of answers for humanity. This may extend to holding outdated perspectives on AESOPs; they may see you as giving in to a fad, or misusing medication if it is prescribed to help. At times, you may experience a subtle or perhaps not-so-subtle pattern of discrimination if you are choosing to deal with your SOP through acknowledging it openly or trying medication. Beware of allowing yourself to feel "less than" others in these cases, and remember to check in with more than one

AESOP=Adults Experiencing Special Operating Problems

source before adopting another's views.

Tools for the Non-Traditionally Minded

Explore your past experiences:

What has spirituality meant to you? Did your SOP prevent you from learning concepts that were presented at home, Bible study, or school? To what or whom do you turn when things seem hopeless? Allow yourself to explore these thoughts and feelings on paper or with a tape recorder.

Pay attention to what brings you peace:

Do feelings of well-being and love come to you when you're walking in nature, watching children play, sitting quietly in a sanctuary? Allowing your spirituality to express itself isn't limited to one formal place or action.

Consider what believing in a Higher Power could provide for you:

First, let's broaden the concept of a Higher Power. According to varying belief systems, this power could be someone or something outside of yourself such as God, the Holy Father, the Trinity, Allah, Yahweh or other entities. In some religious beliefs, this power is considered to be within a person, rather than existing separately as an outside force. But no matter what form your belief in a greater power takes, it gives you someone or something that provides the idea of unwavering support. Beyond that, it holds you to some form of personal accountability. Having a way to deal with your problems by using a Higher Power provides relief and builds a sense of peace and calm, which can all be in short supply for the AESOP.

Look into alternative spiritual practices:

Consider attending a devotional singing group, a Buddhist meditation ceremony, a weekend spiritual retreat. As Adults with SOP we are sometimes reluctant or hesitant to try something new, even though it may turn out wonderfully well. Consider taking a risk in the area of spiritual growth.

Talk to other Adults with SOP about their spiritual beliefs:

It helps to open up and share ideas and beliefs with other AESOPs. With the wide variety of resources available in your community, you may learn about some spiritual opportunities in your area that you never even knew existed.

Consider a 12-Step program:

The 12-Step approach offers a structured systematic program which has as one of its main tenets the need to embrace some sort of a Higher Power. The nature of the Higher Power is left open to a wide range of interpretation. 12-Step programs are usually centered on a specific topic (such as alcoholism, co-dependence, or overeating), but the steps and traditions of the program can affect each area of your life. By working through the twelve steps, many people have found a way to increase self-discipline, consistently work on self-betterment, and develop camaraderie with people very much like themselves. In the 12-Step program, an important facet is the development of a relationship with a person of your choice called a sponsor. This sponsor is usually considered to be older and wiser (either emotionally, spiritually, or in life experiences).

12-Step programs tend to evoke strong emotions in participants. Some AESOPs say a 12-Step program is the only way to go; some object to the structure and find meetings offensive. If you haven't had any 12-Step experience, don't be afraid to try out a meeting or two and decide for yourself.

> "Learn to get in touch with the silence within yourself and know that everything in this life has a purpose."
> -*Elisabeth Kubler-Ross*

AESOP=Adults Experiencing Special Operating Problems

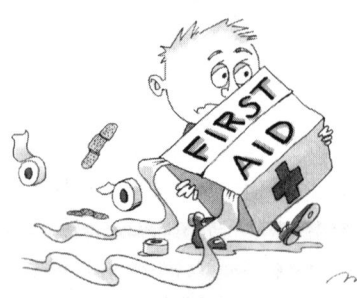

Need More First Aid?

If you feel like other areas of your life also need to be brought into balance, see:
Balance in Life in Chapter 28.

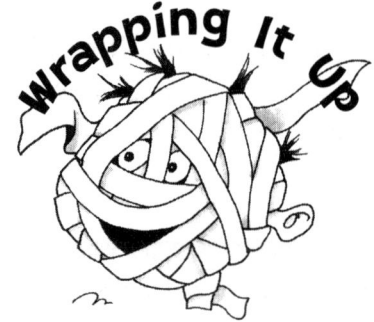

- As AESOPs, we may have developed belief systems that are not in the mainstream of spirituality.

★ The definition of spirituality can easily be expanded to include both traditional and non-traditional sources of strength and support.

- If you are traditionally minded and want to explore your spirituality, there are tools to help.

- If you are non-traditionally minded and yet find yourself wanting to explore what spirituality is for you, there are a number of alternatives to consider.

- No matter who we are, having a spiritual belief system that fits our needs will increase our sense of peace and grounding in life.

> "As humans, we can trace the need for spirituality back to our earliest times. This suggests that spirituality is a necessary part of the human condition for health, both physically and mentally."
> -Joan and Denise

Co-Occurring Conditions

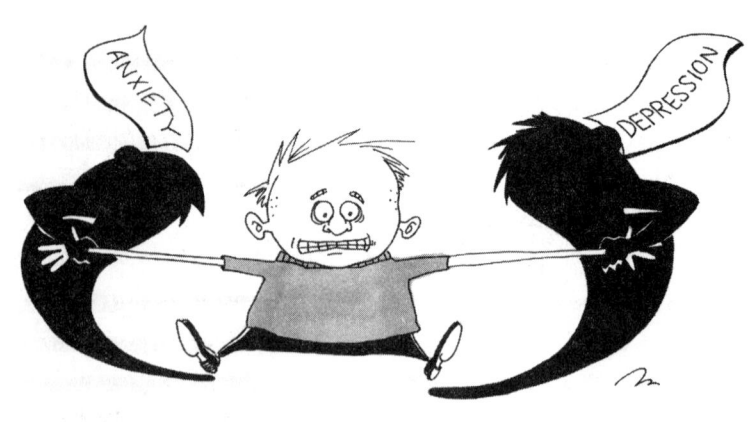

Chapter 35

What You Need To Know

Much of the professional literature uses the term "co-occurring" or "co-morbid" along with Attention Deficit Disorder (ADD), Obsessive Compulsive Disorder (OCD), depression, and rage disorders. While the term "co-morbid" may seem rather formidable, conjuring up thoughts of some kind of life-threatening illness, let us explain it in simple terms. All co-occurring or co-morbid means is that you can have ADD, or OCD, *and* something else at the same time.

For many years the search was on for the "one" gene that caused ADD, or OCD as well as the other disorders. Over the years, our understanding of genetics and genetic complexity has evolved; research

> "The only normal people are the ones you don't know very well."
> -Joe Ancis

now tells us that special operating problems do not come from one single gene, but

AESOP=Adults Experiencing Special Operating Problems

rather a combination of genes. Thus, it is not surprising that with any of these disorders, many adults also have a smattering of something else in the mix.

Some common co-occurring conditions are: anxiety disorders, depression, obsessive compulsive disorders, intermittent rage disorders, and learning disabilities. Be aware that there are actually many more possibilities as well. To be technical, the diagnosis is defined by the primary or most prominent symptom. Thus if a person has major symptoms of ADD, and just a touch of depression, the diagnosis would be ADD with a co-occurring condition of depression. On the other hand, if depression is causing the major amount of problems in an adult's life, then the diagnosis

> *"There are risks and costs to a program of action, but they are far less than the long-range risks and costs of comfortable inactions."*
> —John F. Kennedy

Chapter 35 • Co-Occurring Conditions

would be depression with a co-occurring ADD condition.

So what? Why is the terminology regarding co-occurring conditions important? Actually, for two reasons. One, this terminology is appearing with more and more regularity in the professional literature. Understanding it makes it seem less overwhelming and more manageable. Secondly, the diagnosis itself often dictates the medication that is prescribed as well as the coping techniques that will be effective. For example, let's take an adult with an ADD diagnosis and a co-occurring condition of an anxiety disorder. Stimulant medications are the medications of choice for ADD. They would not be given for an anxiety disorder. However, the designation of the anxiety disorder as a "side disorder" or co-occurring disorder includes the very real possibility that a stimulant medication, as well as an anti-anxiety agent, might be appropriate and might work on the myriad of symptoms. Coping techniques need to be fine-tuned to include those typically used for the ADD adult, with some other tools added to help with the anxiety disorder.

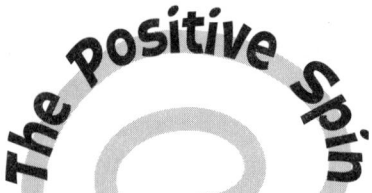
The Positive Spin

As genetic theory is evolving, we now know that special operating problems are often part of a bigger "genetic swirl" that brings in bits and pieces of other conditions. This is good news because it may allow for the possibility of fine-tuning your coping strategies.

Broaden your view! Your own diagnosis may not stand alone, but may be accompanied by "a little bit of this and a little bit of that." Realizing this may make it easier to individualize your treatment, whether that treatment encompasses one or more medications or a variety of coping techniques.

Techniques

List the various traits that cause you difficulty:

Write your Special Operating Problems in a column on paper. Ask yourself if they separate into one or more related categories. Are they consistent over time, or do they come and go? Are they severe enough to cause you real problems or are they just minor annoyances?

> "When we talk to God, we're praying. When God talks to us, we're schizophrenic." –Lily Tomlin

Read books about your primary problem that also include information about co-occurring conditions:

Bookstores can be overwhelming and full of confusing titles. Focusing will allow you to narrow your search. Compare your traits with the various conditions so that you can begin to identify any related diagnoses.

Be aware of misdiagnosing yourself:

Reading just one article, taking a simple test or comparing notes with friends can lead you down the wrong path. Withhold judgment until you have consulted several sources.

AESOP=Adults Experiencing Special Operating Problems

Be aware of misdiagnosis by a professional:

Some professionals are still not adept at recognizing the many facets of co-occurring conditions. Remember, it hasn't been until recently that the overlap between conditions or the concept of co-occurrence has been understood. This misunderstanding is more likely to occur if you are having a conversation about your symptoms with an internist, family practitioner, or gynecologist. They may be seeing only one facet of your profile. If you are sensing that you are dealing with a layering of symptoms, it is very possible that you will need to take the initiative and ask for a referral to a psychiatrist. It is important to realize that seeing a psychiatrist in no sense means that you are "crazy." It simply means that your combination

> "Never stay in treatment with a doctor who thinks that you can't get better."
> -Andrew Weil, MD

of symptoms needs the attention of a specialist. The parallel here is asking for a referral from your primary care physician to a specialist to treat your knee injury. A specialist knows the intricacies of treatment.

Seek appropriate professional help:

If your special operating problems and co-occurring conditions require more than coping techniques alone, find someone who specializes in your primary SOP and can deal with co-occurring conditions. This can be the psychiatrist we mentioned above. Interview professionals about their approaches to co-occurring conditions. You are looking for two things in this conversation. One is their understanding of the subject. The second, and equally as important, is their willingness to treat your questions with respect.

Special note:

If you are calling a psychiatrist it is not at all unusual to be told by the receptionist that you must make an appointment to even ask your questions. Don't let this put you off. Be prepared to treat the first session as an opportunity for you to evaluate the psychiatrist using the suggestions above.

Recognize that you may require a "medication cocktail":

The newest medical information coming from national conferences indicates that we are moving away from prescribing just one medication to treat SOP. Instead, the trend is to see more than one medication prescribed in small, balanced doses with each medication designated to treat a specific symptom. Medical treatment has been expanded to recognize that the more talented the mixologist, the more effective the treatment. Another trend is to see a combination of Eastern medicine (acupuncture and herbs) used along with Western medicine.

Obviously, if two practitioners are supplying treatment, they must coordinate their efforts.

Learn to use specific coping techniques for specific problems:

Once you have identified your co-occurring conditions, see related chapters in this book to expand your repertoire of coping tools. This book is

> "One doesn't discover new lands without consenting to lose sight of the shore for a very long time."
> —*Andre Gide*

meant to be a quick and easy reference and to provide specific techniques. If the first one doesn't work, don't be afraid to try the next suggestion. For example, let's suppose that you have identified elements of Attention Deficit Disorder coupled with an overlaying depression. As you examine your own brand of ADD, you find that your main difficulty has to do with concentration and inability to focus, especially when you are sitting in long boring business meetings. It really doesn't seem to give you much trouble in more interesting settings, such as in conversations with your co-workers. One coping technique for business meetings would be to become an avid note-taker. You may never read the notes again, but the act of writing in itself will allow you to focus. It will also give the illusion that you are very interested in the meeting content.

Now you must deal with a coping technique for your overlay of depression. In your reading you find that cardiovascular exercise often alleviates depression. You try it and find that it works well for you. This means that you will need to be religious about a regular program of running, swimming, or biking three or four times a week.

> "It requires a great deal of inexperience to be beyond the reach of anxiety."
> -20,000 Quotes and Quips

Enlighten family members:

Family members are often alarmed when a multiple diagnosis is given. They become even more frightened when more than one medication is prescribed. People unfamiliar with SOP may perceive the medication cocktail as drug overuse, rather than a highly specialized form of treatment. Educate your family. This is a vital part of overcoming their resistance and enlisting their help.

Chapter 35 • Co-Occurring Conditions

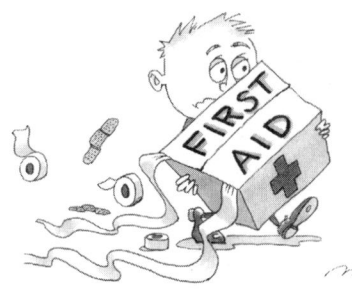

Need More First Aid?

If you need information on depression or other mood-related concerns, see:
Moods in Chapter 16 or Depression in Chapter 17

If your co-occurring condition includes problems with chemical dependency, see:
Addictions in Chapter 33.

If your special operating problem is colliding with menopause symptoms, see:
Menopause in Chapter 36.

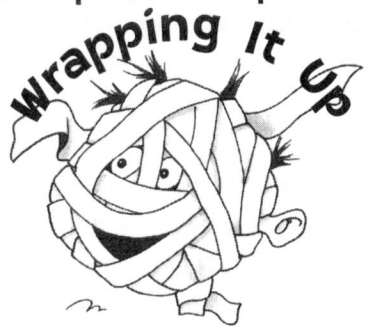

- "Co-occurring" or "co-morbidity" are clinical terms

that simply mean that more than one condition is present at the same time.

- If you have the genes for one condition, you may also have the predisposition to another.

- A combination of medication(s) and coping techniques will often be needed when more than one condition is present.

- Frequently, medication "cocktails" are prescribed and represent effective treatment, not drug overuse.

- Sometimes a combination of Western and Eastern medicine is used.

- The most important key to understanding co-occurring conditions is educating yourself and your family about the disorders.

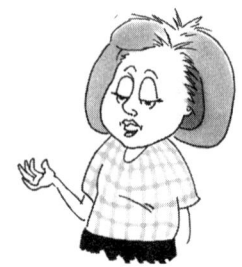

Chapter 35 • Co-Occurring Conditions

> "Special Operating Problems are often part of a bigger 'genetic swirl' that bring in bits and pieces of other conditions. This is good news, because it may allow for the possibility of fine-tuning your coping strategies."
>
> *-Joan and Denise*

AESOP=Adults Experiencing Special Operating Problems

Menopause

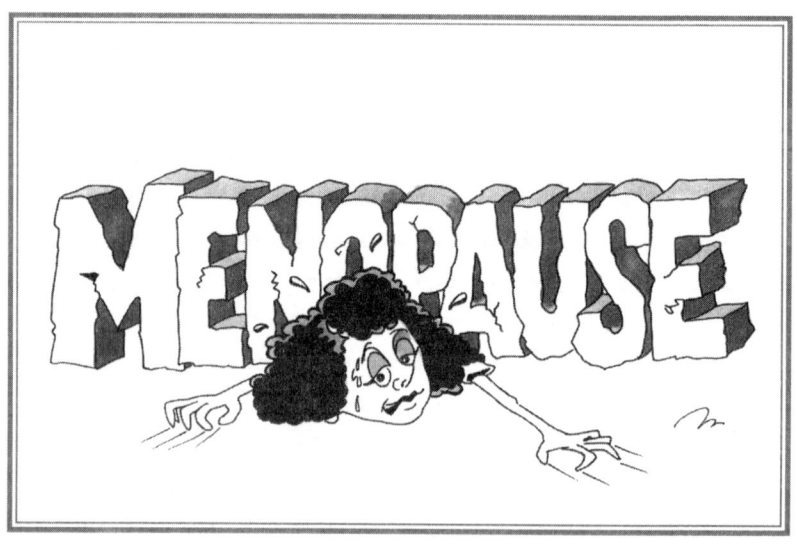

Chapter 36

What You Need To Know

Menopause happens! After moving through adolescence and childbearing, menopause is the last monumental physical and hormonal shift that a woman's body will face. It is also the least understood phase of a woman's life. A mountain of knowledge is available in all bookstores about the child-rearing years. New mothers talk unendingly about the changes pregnancy brings to their bodies and spirits. But what about menopause? It is either spoken about in hushed tones or used as a topic for jokes. Any books on the subject are typically found in one tiny section of the bookstore. For AESOPs, it is nearly impossible to find anything substantial about the correlation between menopause and the symptoms of their SOP.

For a woman who carries the genetic disposition to difficulties with SOP but hasn't been much affected by them, this means that suddenly, after a productive, fulfilling life, she may change radically at

AESOP=Adults Experiencing Special Operating Problems

menopause. For her, menopause may bring changes that are more severe than those her friends of the same age experience. She may begin to feel a little more fuzzy in the brain. Her memory may begin to slip. Moods, depression, and anger may escalate. Her co-workers, friends, or family may accuse her of being totally unreasonable or impossible to deal with when she thinks she is feeling and acting as rationally as ever.

If her pattern of difficulties with SOP has been more pronounced throughout life, she can expect the hormonal shifts at menopause to kick all of her symptoms up to a new level. This is often frightening, because while she is aware that she is not functioning as well as before, finding a professional or physician who understands how strongly the hormones can escalate all kinds of symptoms, let alone treats them successfully, is extremely difficult.

> "I have bursts of being a lady, but it doesn't last long." *-Shelley Winters*

Menopause symptoms may take an unexpected turn. A woman's self-esteem may plummet because her memory is faulty and she finds that she is forgetting appointments or promises to her best friend or spouse. She may rather abruptly decide she hates her husband or job and begin to consider life alone on Bora Bora. These trends can be scary if the woman with SOP doesn't see them for what they are: simply the exacerbation of her SOP due to menopause.

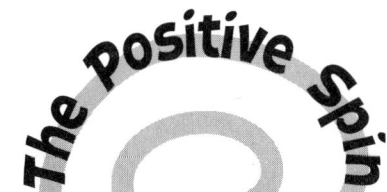

The Positive Spin

Stop doubting yourself! If things have gone smoothly for years and suddenly you are experiencing the symptoms listed above, realize that a flare-up of problems at menopause is very normal. Even though you will find almost nothing in the literature connecting AESOPs and menopause, even if your treating physician tells you that he or she is not aware of any correlation, even if your family,

AESOP=Adults Experiencing Special Operating Problems

friends, or co-workers act as though you are crazy, trust yourself. Insist that your AESOP symptoms at this time of life be treated with just as much attention and care as those of an adolescent with SOP. In adolescence, it is common knowledge that the need for medication may be at its highest point. In fact, it is not at all unusual for symptoms to increase at adolescence to the point that medication is needed even if it was never needed before and might not be needed after. This is also true at menopause. Be resolute, and insist you get treatment that will stabilize you through this difficult period.

Techniques
Support Systems

Find a friend:

Other women who can support you through menopause (AESOPs themselves if at all possible) are invaluable. It is

Chapter 36 • Menopause

so wonderful to hear someone reaffirm you by saying, "Oh yes, I feel that way too!"

Use information as support:

Attack the subject of AESOPs and menopause as you would any other problem. Research the subject individually by going to the library, the bookstore, using the Internet, and attending any local conferences related to your own specific type of SOP.

Consider the Web:

For most women at the age of menopause, using the Web may seem as foreign to them as speaking another language. Actually, the Web is often an incredibly helpful avenue of communication that will allow you to link up with other women through chat rooms or email. Once you are comfortable navigating the Web, you will find it an unending source of up-to-date information. As an added bonus, you are often able to tap into sources aimed at professionals which won't be available in print for six months to a year.

Find a therapist:

This professional must have a special set of qualifications.

He or she must be well-versed about all stages of working with AESOPs, be able to speak clearly and knowledgeably about the connection between AESOPs and menopause, and be willing to advocate for you with your physician, if necessary.

Emotional Relief

Get a grip!

Yes, menopause is a pain in the neck, but you made it through adolescence, child bearing, and you will make it through this last passage. This is yet another time in life that, as a woman, you need to be strong. You can do it.

Consider writing:

If you have gotten relief in the past from journal writing as you moved through a difficult period, try it again.

Take a trip:

Sometimes getting away from your job, your husband, your family, and your house will give you a breath of fresh air and some clarity. Be sure that those around you understand that you are not just running away from life, but are trying to take better care of yourself.

Distract yourself:

We talk often in this book about balance in life. At menopause, balance is vital. Be sure that you maintain a balance between work, play, and spirituality.

> "From birth to age 18, a girl needs good parents, from 18 to 35 she needs good looks, from 35 to 55 she needs a good personality, and from 55 on, she needs cash."
> —*Sophie Tucker*

Develop a passion in life:

If you have been a "good" wife and a mother for years or an extremely responsible member in the workplace, and you are feeling cranky and icky at this stage, let your mind explore your options. Maybe this is the time to take up long distance running or race walking, learn how to quilt, enroll in medical school or a Ph.D. program. You will know you have arrived at the stage of having a passion when you find yourself saying something like "Well, I'm really upset, but at least I can go walking this afternoon." A passion is something that excites you, makes you happy when you think about it, and takes you over the rough spots.

Medical Relief

Investigate medication for menopause:

It is important to stabilize the body chemistry as much as possible, so hormonal replacement therapy and/or antidepressants should be considered. These are often prescribed at menopause and may lessen symptoms. The decision to use hormone replacement therapy involves assessing your family history and risk factors; you'll need to do your own research along with obtaining medical advice.

Consider medication for your symptoms:

Whether you have been on medication prior to menopause or not, if problems with SOP run in your family, you may need treatment with some type of stimulant medication to help clear the fuzzy thinking

Chapter 36 • Menopause

and alleviate some of the memory lapses. You may also need an anti-depressant at this time. Realize that the newer class of anti-depressants (called SSRI's) such as Prozac, Zoloft, and Paxil, as well as other medications such as Serzone, Effexor and Wellbutrin allow more serotonin to remain available in the brain. Although they are

> "My after forty face felt far more comfortable than anything I lived with previously. Self-confidence was a powerful beauty-potion; I looked better because I felt better. Failure and grief as well as success and love had served me well. Finally, I was tapping into that most hard-won of youth dues: wisdom."
>
> *-Nancy Collins*

AESOP=Adults Experiencing Special Operating Problems

sold under the designation of "anti-depressants," they also work on anger and rage. If you are prickly, hostile, furious with life, prone to rage, or if you are weepy and sad, consider trying an anti-depressant. These can often be used in conjunction with other medications.

Arrange for a reality check:

Target a sympathetic friend who is willing to give you some honest feedback on your functioning ability as well as your moods, depression and anger. Don't use a husband or child to perform this function. If you are angry, you won't believe them anyway.

Pick a physician with care:

This is a time to interview several physicians about their medical expertise in treating menopause, especially if you are an Adult with SOP. If you don't come away with a good feeling that a physician understands the seriousness of your concerns and can provide intelligent information about the correlation between your symptoms and menopause, don't delay; find someone else.

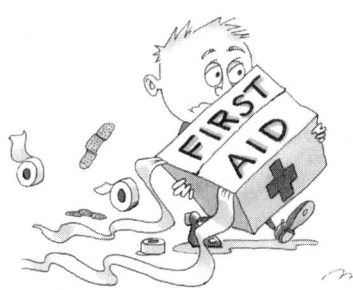

Need More First Aid?

If papers around the house seem to be accumulating faster than ever before, see:
Chapter 7 on Clutter.

If life has seemed flat with more low spots than high spots, check out:
Chapter 17 on Depression.

If you have been a dutiful wife and mother all your life with little thought for yourself, read:
Balance in Life in Chapter 28.

If you feel that your body is falling apart, see:
Chapter 29 on Diet and Chapter 30 on Exercise.

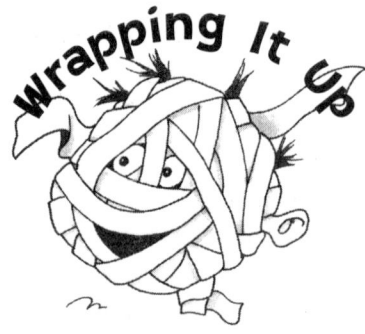

Wrapping It Up

- Menopause is probably the least understood phase of a woman's life.

- For a woman with SOP, menopause has the possibility of accelerating all of the symptoms that have been well under control for years. Worse yet, if symptoms haven't been under control, menopause can be expected to kick everything up to a new level.

- To make it more difficult, little is written about the correlation between AESOPs and the escalation of symptoms at menopause.

- Understanding coping techniques that will help you through this time is crucial. Developing support systems and finding emotional relief as well as professional help is vitally important.

Chapter 36 • Menopause

● Be resolute and insist that you get support and treatment to help stabilize you during this difficult period.

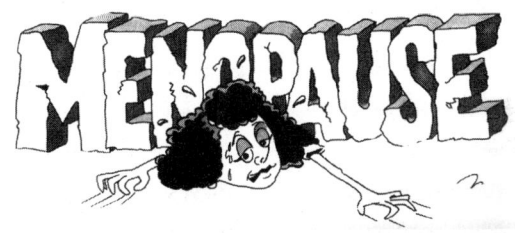

MENOPAUSE

> "New mothers talk unendingly about the changes pregnancy brings to their bodies and spirits. But what about menopause? It is either spoken about in hushed tones or used as a topic for jokes."
>
> *-Joan and Denise*

Bibliography

Brilliant, A. <u>I Have Abandoned My Search For Truth, and Am Now Looking for a Good Fantasy.</u> Santa Barbara, CA: Woodbridge Press Publishing Company, 1997.

Brown Jr., J.B. <u>A Father's Book of Wisdom.</u> Tennessee: Rutledge Hill Press, 1988.

Brown, Jr., H.J. <u>Life's Little Treasure Book on Wisdom.</u> Nashville, Tennessee: Rutledge Hill Press, 1991, 93, 94.

Brown, Jr., H.J. <u>Life's Little Treasure Book on Success.</u> Nashville, Tennessee: Rutledge Hill Press, 1991, 92, 93, 94.

Brown, Jr., H.J. <u>Life's Little Treasure Book on Hope.</u> Nashville, Tennessee: Rutledge Hill Press, 1991, 92, 93, 94.

Byrne, R., Editor. <u>The 2548 Best Things Anybody Ever Said.</u> New York, NY: Galahad Books, 1996.

Bibliography

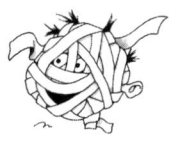

Byrne, R. <u>The 637 Best Things Anybody Ever Said.</u>
New York, NY: Ballantine Books, 1982.

Carne, P. <u>Out of the Shadows: Understanding Sexual Addiction.</u>
Hazelden Information and Educational Services, 1992.

Corman, C. and Greenberg, L. <u>All You Ever Wanted To Know About Attention Deficits But Didn't Know Whom To Ask...</u> Los Alamitos, CA:
Universal Attention Disorders, Inc, 1997.

Eisen, A. <u>Go For The Gold: Thoughts on Achieving Your Personal Best.</u> Kansas City, Missouri: Andrews and McMeel, Universal Press Syndicate Company, 1995.

Eisen, A. <u>Believing in Ourselves: The Wisdom of Women.</u>
Kansas City, Missouri: Andrews and McMeel,
Universal Press Syndicate Company, 1995.

Esar, E. <u>20,000 Quips and Quotes.</u>
New York, NY: Barnes and Noble, Inc., 1995.

Bibliography

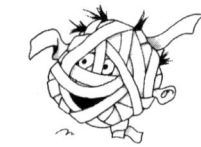

Frank, L.R. <u>Quotationary.</u>
    New York, NY: Random House, 1999.

Larned, M. <u>Stone Soup for the World.</u>
    New York, NY: MJF Books, 1998.

Lazear, J. <u>Meditations for Men Who Do Too Much.</u>
    New York, NY: Simon and Schuster, 1992.

McWilliams, P. <u>The Portable DO IT!</u>
    Los Angeles, CA: Prelude Press, 1993.

McWilliams, P. <u>The Portable Life 101.</u>
    Los Angeles, CA: Prelude Press, 1992.

Mieder, W. <u>Prentice-Hall Encyclopedia of World Proverbs.</u>
    New York, NY: MJF Books, 1986.

Peale, N.V. <u>My Favorite Quotations.</u>
    New York, NY: Harper, San Francisco, 1990.

Bibliography

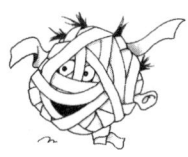

Quotable Women: <u>A Collection of Shared Thoughts.</u>
    Philadelphia, Pennsylvania:
    Running Press Book Publishers, 1989, 1994.

Schaef, A. <u>365 Mediations Reflections and Restoratives for Women Who Do Too Much</u>. New York, NY:
    Workman Publishing, 1999.

Shanahan, J.M., Editor <u>The Most Brilliant Thoughts of All Time.</u>
    New York, NY: Cliff Street Books, 1999.

Toms, M. (Interviewer); Buckley, M. (Editor). <u>Wise Words: Perennial Wisdom from the New Dimensions Radio Series.</u> Carlsbad, GA: Hay House, Inc, 1997.

Whiter, B. and Pinkney, M. <u>Pocket Positives.</u>
    Australia: Five Miles Press Pty. Ltd, 1997.

Zadra, D. <u>To Your Success.</u>
    Hong Kong: Compendium Inc, 1997.

A

ability, intellectual, 50, 247
abuse, 484, 486
abuse, alcohol, 14, 350, 484-485, 506
abuse, drug, 234, 475, 485, 521-522
abuse, substance, 3, 230, 485, 487, 490, 492, 494
academics, 378, 402, 410
abusive behavior, 492
accommodations, 161, 362, 409
activities, high intensity(see exercise)
activities, low intensity (see exercise)
activity, physical, 39, 41, 53, 115, 185, 218, 228, 233, 245, 251, 264-265, 286, 386, 413, 438, 440-452, 456, 467, 471-472, 481, 483, 493, 520, 536
acupuncture, 220, 234-235, 518
ADA, Americans with Disabilities Act, 159-161, 360-364
ADD in the workplace, 160-161, 270, 363, 532
addiction, 14, 339, 422, 476-480, 483-484, 488-493, 495

addiction, gambling, 489, 493
addiction, sexual, 339, 489, 491-492
adolescent, 376, 383, 387-388, 529
adrenaline, 92, 269
adulthood, 375
aggression, 16
alcohol abuse, 24, 358, 492-493, 514
allergies, 221-222
anger, 16, 181, 227, 242, 261-272, 276, 299, 304, 309, 368, 503, 527, 535
antidepressants, 233, 350, 488, 533-535
anxiety, 4, 158, 181, 187, 295, 396, 512-514, 520
athletes, 273

B

biochemical, 20, 232, 245, 262, 269, 272, 286, 339, 381, 384, 475, 478, 486, 495
boredom, 129-130, 138, 355, 368, 450
brain, 5, 17, 25, 35, 61, 68, 87, 123-124, 132-133, 218, 221, 224, 231, 235, 265, 308, 319, 361, 467, 486, 527, 534

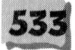

Index

brainstorm, 40, 50-51, 61, 83, 159, 357, 378
breathing techniques, 22, 37-39, 198, 208, 219, 267, 308, 378, 404, 432, 447, 466, 468, 531
bulimia, 489

C

caffeine, 14, 483
career, 10, 13, 23, 28, 35, 39, 43, 47-49, 59, 61-62, 66, 69, 73, 75, 79, 81, 91, 101-103, 115, 117-118, 124, 129-130, 136, 138, 145, 159-160, 165-166, 171, 174, 176, 185, 188, 196-197, 199-202, 205, 211, 213, 228, 231, 236, 251-252, 260, 263, 269, 272, 276, 284, 287, 289-290, 298, 301, 304, 313, 316, 328, 331, 338, 341, 345-347, 349, 354-358, 360-369, 371, 373, 377, 380, 383, 391, 393, 396-397, 404, 410-412, 415, 417, 420, 422-424, 428, 441, 443, 445, 449, 455-458, 465, 469, 475, 481, 485-486, 492, 507, 513, 519, 532, 535

Disabled Student Center, 162, 164, 394
chiropractor, 235
chocolate, 435
cigarettes, 477, 484
centering, 39, 236, 506
chemistry, 5
co-workers, 28, 356, 358
childhood, 12, 231, 255, 381, 383, 393
childrearing, 526
classroom, 15, 393, 399-400
cleanliness, 110, 118-120, 300, 414
clutter, 101, 113
coaching, 39, 129, 243, 329, 425
cocktail, medication, 522
cocaine, 486
coffee, 14, 91, 95, 103, 197, 290, 328, 341, 475-476, 482-483
college, 50, 124, 145, 162, 174, 181, 209, 236, 393, 397-402, 406
codependence, 506
cognitive thinking, 224, 228
co-morbidity, 511, 522

compassion, 254, 278
complacency, 71
comprehension, 182, 409-410
concentration, 350, 362, 411, 519
conceptualization, 8, 72, 76, 93-95, 170, 173, 259, 324, 375, 411, 424, 426-427, 478, 504-505, 516
compulsiveness, 3, 61, 106, 295, 415, 489, 511-512
computers, 77, 82, 151, 162-163
co-occurring conditions, 181, 189, 227, 245, 389, 416, 510-520, 522-523
consequences, 11, 45, 54, 110, 132, 170, 178, 185, 187, 285, 299, 304, 379, 383, 388, 466, 486
coping, 10, 17, 92, 98, 107, 115, 136, 142-143, 319, 373, 390, 465, 471, 473, 513-514, 517, 519-520, 522, 524, 537
counseling, 40, 162, 164, 181, 236, 376, 402-403
cravings, 222
cues, memory, 77, 105, 109, 152, 264, 286, 317-318, 320, 332, 355, 365, 368, 446, 527-528, 534

D

dangerous activities, 37, 233, 247, 405, 486
daytimer, 75, 82
deadlines, 401, 414
defensiveness, 256
degree, graduate , 361, 393, 416
denial, 276, 384
depression, 3-5, 10, 12-13, 26-27, 33, 111, 119, 180-181, 188-189, 191-192, 225, 230-236, 238, 240-248, 259, 263, 276, 281, 338, 341, 371, 416, 433, 438, 441, 445, 448, 470, 489, 511-513, 519-521, 527, 535-536
despair, 45, 213, 373
disability, 159, 161-163, 165, 360, 364, 394, 398-400, 406-407, 409
discipline, 274, 399, 421
disease, 477-478
Obsessive Compulsive Disorder (OCD), 365, 376, 511
Oppositional Defiant Disorder

Index

(ODD)*****
disorders, anxiety, 513-514
disorders, depressive, 5, 12, 188, 245, 338
disorganization, 295, 372
distractibility, 80, 83-84, 121, 138, 148, 161, 361, 400
DNA, 477
dopamine, 195
drug abuse *(see abuse, drug)*

E

eating disorders *(see also addiction, food)* 489
education, vocational, 364, 397
ejaculation, 350
emotion, 5, 103, 108, 189, 217, 220, 224-225, 227, 239-240, 262-263, 271-272, 275, 279, 282, 324, 336, 338, 350, 360, 427, 507-508, 531, 537
empathy, 374
emotional abuse *(see abuse, emotional)*
employee, 160, 360
employers, 176

energy, 323, 468
endorphins, 218
environment, work, 118, 160
enrolling in school, 395, 401, 416, 532
estrogen, 448
exams, 252
exercise, 39, 41, 53, 115, 185, 218, 228, 233, 245, 251, 264-265, 286, 386-387, 413, 421, 438, 440-452, 456, 467, 471-472, 481, 483, 493, 520, 536
exhaustion, 288
extroversion, 323, 332

F

family, 5, 277, 294, 304-305, 425
father, 5, 189, 505
fighting, 232, 248, 475
focusing, 270, 431, 446, 483, 515
food addiction *(see addiction, food)*
finances, handling, 125, 150-151, 157, 173
forgetfulness, 85, 284-285, 319, 528
frustration, 18, 30, 135, 268, 270,

291, 294-295, 355, 465

G

gambling (see addiction, gambling)
genetics, 301
guilt, 73, 89, 116, 185, 256, 387
grieving, 275-277
gynecologist, 516

H

habits, 214-215, 239, 242, 285, 289-290, 307, 317, 319, 404, 435, 450, 476, 482, 490
headaches, 221, 267
helplessness, 477
herbs, 219, 228, 233-234, 265, 456
heroin, 486
holistic medicine, 234
homeopathic remedies, 219
hormones, 341, 383, 526-527, 533
hyperactivity, 15, 221, 338, 463-465, 468, 471, 473
hypoactive, 15, 338, 464, 468-469
hypnosis, 39

I

impatience, 125, 324

impulses, 11, 53-54, 122-124, 126, 128, 130-133, 177, 207, 214, 287, 350, 383-386, 492
inattention, 284, 316, 400
inactivity, 441
inconsiderateness, 195, 284, 299
inconsistency, 14, 115, 117, 355, 371, 432, 443
Individuals with Disabilities Education Act, 26, 33, 103, 105-106, 110, 148, 162, 190, 231, 301, 319, 346, 348, 498-499, 505
insomnia, 342
inspiration, 18, 105
instructor, 404-407, 411-412, 414
intelligence, 324, 387, 427, 535
instructor, teacher, 404-407, 411-412, 414
introversion, 323
in-to-me-see, 313, 332

J

job *(see career)*

L

language, written, 407, 409

lateness, 195-196, 200-203, 289, 355, 460
Civil Rights Law, 161
learning, 11, 159, 162-165, 191, 218, 280, 378-379, 394-395, 398-400, 405, 407, 415-417, 456, 504, 512
lethargy, 445, 448
loneliness, 61, 241, 264
loving, 78, 253, 492
lovemaking, 128
lying, 290, 382, 384-385, 455

M

maturing, 128
management, time, 31, 68, 70, 72-74, 76, 78-80, 82, 84, 86, 88, 98, 141, 203, 214, 367, 413, 428, 449
marijuana, 14, 475-476
marriage, 387
massage, 235
master's degree, 393, 416
medication, 486
meditating, 326
menstruation, 217
mentors, 40, 125-127, 190, 209, 254, 425
medicine, 219-220, 228, 235, 518, 523
medicine, Eastern, 220, 235, 518, 523
medicine, Western, 220, 228, 518
meditation, 38-39, 223, 225, 235, 456, 468, 481, 501, 506
memory, 77, 105, 109, 152, 264, 286, 317-318, 320, 332, 355, 365, 368, 446, 527-528, 534
men, 335
message, 213, 264, 287-288, 351, 365, 374, 490
minerals, 218, 220
misdiagnosis, 515-516
misunderstood, 284, 347
moodiness, 13, 217
mothers, 526, 538

N

neatness, compulsive, 300
nightmares, 395
nutrition, 432, 466, 472

O

Office of Civil Rights*****
organization, 9, 58-66, 68, 141,

Index

238, 242, 501
organization, 65-66, 68, 87, 102, 118, 141, 192
orgasm, 350
over-arousal, 16
over-committing, 424
over-dieting, 431
over-eating, 431, 433, 489, 507
over-reaction, 382
over-spending, 124
overwhelm, 14, 24, 26, 28, 30, 32, 86, 97, 111-112, 141, 191, 367, 428

P

parent, 387
painkilling, 485
partnerships, 341
passion, 210, 532-533
pathological, 385-386
pharmaceuticals, 396
pharmacist, 234, 350
physician, 233-234, 247, 414, 456, 480, 487-488, 517, 527-528, 531, 535
pills, diet, 476, 484-485

planning, 115, 132, 412
pot *(see marijuana)*
practitioner, family, 235, 516, 518
prayer, 223, 468, 501, 515
predisposed, 5, 296, 455, 462, 522
pregnancy, 526, 538
preoccupation, 267
prescriptions, 199, 233-235, 350, 456, 475, 483-484, 487-488, 491, 493, 503, 513, 518, 521-522, 533
problems, learning disabilities, 11, 394, 415
problems, mood, 223
program, 12-Step, 237, 488, 506-508
productivity, 117-118, 161, 187, 200, 227, 359, 366, 422, 457-458, 470, 526
professor, 164, 409
psychiatry, 4, 233, 247, 488, 517-518
psychologists, 4, 224
psychostimulants, 350

R

rage, 3, 13, 16, 262, 264, 272, 309, 338, 351, 365, 511-512, 535

recovery programs, 393, 416
registration, early or priority, 154, 404
regret, 275
Rehabilitation Act, 407
rehabilitation, 364, 407, 490
relapse, 290, 292, 480, 489
relaxation, 35, 37-39, 116, 129, 137, 202, 235, 344, 386, 456, 476
religion, 223, 497
re-prioritizing, 81
reprogram, 39, 253
testing, scantron, 163, 395
resentment, 200, 323, 344, 366
retirement, 126, 154, 158-159, 174, 176
rigidity, 497
romance, 372, 387, 389
rudeness, 195, 284, 348

S

schizophrenic, 515
school, highschool experience, 181, 236, 238, 398, 400-401
shoolwork, 110
secretaries, 78

self-acceptance, 469
self-awareness, 26
self-berating, 470
self-betterment, 507
self-confidence, 534
self-control, 62
self-correction, self-discipline, 507
self-doubt, 388
self-esteem, 200, 251, 262, 528
self-expression, 332
self-help, 16, 22, 224
self-hypnosis, 456
self-management, 62
self-medicating, 350, 483, 485-487, 491, 493
self-monitoring, 264, 266, 272
serotonin, 231, 534
sex, 313-314, 330-332, 334-353, 389, 460, 491, 494
sexuality, 351-352, 491
sexual addiction *(see addiction, sexual)*
shame, 55, 98, 102, 245, 249-255, 257, 259-260, 263, 281, 476, 478, 485-486

skills, social, 296
sleep, 48, 198-200, 203-204, 223, 239, 241, 264-265, 271, 285-286, 298, 342-343, 380, 382, 413, 420, 443, 453-462, 471
society, 15, 290, 497
solutions, 3-4, 18, 40, 46, 50-51, 55, 141, 159, 161, 232, 248, 280, 320, 324-325, 333, 356-359, 369, 380, 406, 411
speed, 36, 244, 324, 464, 466, 486
spelling, 400
spontaneity, impulsivity, 60, 301
spouse, 40, 87, 93, 126, 128, 262, 286, 302, 307, 309, 345, 387, 459, 481, 528
spontaneous, 60
stabilizers, 199, 219, 350, 475, 478-479, 529, 533, 538
specialist, 39, 219, 223, 398, 400, 517
shoplifting, 383
stereotypes, 11
stimulants, 199, 480, 488, 513, 533
stimulation, 119, 128-129, 135, 297, 387, 483
stress, 29, 31, 34-43, 97, 135, 141-142, 156, 209, 226, 264, 268, 270-271, 286, 298, 307-308, 352, 367, 388, 411, 414-415, 424, 437, 470, 483
student, 162, 164-165, 393-394, 407-408
studying, 411
suffering, 231, 399, 411, 480
supplement, 218, 408
structure, 67, 223, 306, 377, 391, 420, 436, 508
substance, illegal *(see addiction, drug)*

T

teacher, 63, 190, 238-239, 371, 375, 384, 386, 398
temper, 218, 275, 287, 294, 296, 308, 355, 390
therapy, 488
therapy, cognitive, 224, 228
therapy, cognitive, 165, 224, 244, 228, 280, 306, 413, 488, 492
therapy, traditional, 165, 244, 280, 306, 413, 488, 492

Order Form

1. Books:

Quantity   Amount

Tourette Syndrome and Human Behavior
_____ 1S Softback $39.95   _____

Search for the Tourette Syndrome and Human Behavior Genes
_____ 8H Hardback $34.00   _____
_____ 8S Softback $29.95   _____

The Gene Bomb - Does Higher Education and Advanced Technology Accelerate the Selection of Genes for Learning Disorders, ADHD, Addictive and Disruptive Behaviors?
_____ 9H Hardback $29.95   _____
_____ 9S Softback $25.00   _____

RYAN — A Mother's Story of Her Hyperactive-Tourette Syndrome Child
_____ 2S Softback $9.95   _____

What Makes Ryan Tick? A Family's Triumph over TS and ADHD
_____ 10S Softback $14.95   _____

Hi, I'm Adam - A Child's Book about Tourette Syndrome
_____ 4A Softback $4.95   _____

Adam and the Magic Marble
_____ 4B Softback $6.95   _____

Hi, I'm Adam + Adam and the Magic Marble
_____ 4C Both together $11.50   _____

Don't Think About Monkeys - Extraordinary Stories by People with Tourette Syndrome
_____ 6A Softback $12.95   _____

Teaching the Tiger - A Handbook for Individuals Involved in the Education of Students with Attention Deficit Disorder, Tourette Syndrome or Obsessive-Compulsive Disorder
_____ 7A Softback $35.00   _____

A.D.D. Kaleidoscope - The Many Facets of Adult AttentionDeficit Disorder
_____ 8A Softback $24.95 _____

Understanding and Treating the Tourette Syndrome/ADHD Spectrum Disorders by Dr. Comings 8 tapes 10 hrs
_____ 11A $75.00 _____

Dysinhibition Syndrome - How to Handle Anger and Rage in Your Child or Spouse
_____ 12A Softback $24.95 _____

Check-up from the Neck-up - Ensuring Mental Health in the Next Millennium
_____ 13A Softback $19.95 _____

Subtotal for Books _____

2. Tax: California residents please add 8.25% sales tax _____

3. Mailing and Handling:
- ☐ Fourth Class: $4.00 lst item $1.00 each additional item
- ☐ U.P.S. Ground: $6.00 lst item $1.00 each additional item
- ☐ U.P.S. Air: $10.00 lst item $2.00 each additional item _____

Name:_____ **Total** _____

Address: _____

City: _____ State:_____ Zip: _____

Country (if other than U.S.A.): _____

Check Enclosed _____ **or** Visa ___ Mastercard ___

CC# _____ Expiration Date _____

send to: Hope Press P.O.Box 188, Duarte, CA 91009-0188

or Fill out this form with credit card # and FAX it to 626-358-3520

or Order by phone **1-800-321-4039** — 24 hr service

for more details on each book visit our web site: **http://www.hopepress.com**

therapists, 254, 349, 480, 530
sympathy, 110, 213, 240, 279, 366, 380, 404, 535
thrill-seeking, 128
timeout, 267-268, 296, 298, 322, 380, 383-384
tired, 264, 322, 468
toolbox, tools for your, 74, 78, 198
journaling, 277
training, 39, 218, 361, 393, 398, 426
transcripts, 401, 414
transpose, 395
triggers, 13, 17, 77, 145, 222, 226, 262-264, 267, 269, 272, 457, 483, 486
tutor, 51, 165, 280, 408, 411-412
timer, 76, 103, 119, 138, 197-198, 289, 456
tolerance, frustration , 18, 268, 270, 295, 355
treatment, 105, 199, 228, 235, 280, 477-480, 485, 487, 489, 491, 514, 516-518, 521-522, 529, 533, 538

U

under-diagnosis, 27

uniqueness, 73, 202, 500-501
university, 145, 162, 164, 166, 393, 398, 401, 407
unmotivated, 16, 111
unpredictable, 297, 310, 465
vision, tunnel, 52, 197, 379, 425

V

visualization, 268, 313, 427
vitamins, 218, 220, 234, 413
vocational training, 364, 397

W

women, 305, 327-330, 336, 447, 529-530
work *(see career, job)*
workload, 403, 405
workout, 442, 467-468, 481
worry, excessive, 184, 236, 257
writing, 395

Y

yoga, 38, 223, 235, 481

What Reviewers Have Said:

Delightful! Humorous! Yet this little book offers enormous *bites* of serious information and advice to all of the AESOPs of the world. And are we not all AESOPs in one arena or another? Kudos to Joan and Denise.

>Edna D. Copeland, Ph.D.
>Director, National Professional Consortium in Attention Deficit Disorders
>Author of *Attention Please*

Check Up from the Neck Up is a must read for anyone who seeks to improve the quality of their life in the new millennium. Refreshingly alive, filled with humor, inspiration, and practical strategies to make our hectic lives easier. Andrews and Davis provide concrete, easy to implement tools to help deal with common human problems ranging from depression, substance abuse, ADD, to clutter management, stress reduction, relationships issues, money management, and sex. The authors' wisdom comes not only from their educational background, but years of personal and professional experience with the issues that they so compassionately address. Pick this book up for yourself, a friend, or loved one. It's a true gem!

> Wendy Richardson, MA MFT
> Author of *The Link Between ADD &
> Addiction: Getting the Help You Deserve*

This is a book for each one of us. A remarkable book with a wealth of information to aid us in dealing with common life struggles.

> Stephen C. Copps, M.D.
> Director, MCCG Institute for
> Developmental Medicine, Macon, Georgia
> Author of *The Attending Physician*

• • • • • • • • • • • • • • • •
Check Up From the Neck Up

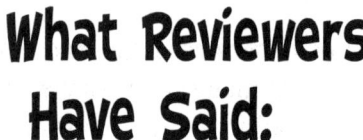

What Reviewers Have Said:

I highly recommend Andrews and Davis' dynamic new book, full of easy to understand and transferable techniques. The topics will start you thinking and give you answers to questions that have long been floating in the back of your mind. There is a banquet of insights that can help you find joy and get ahead in life. The "Positive Spin" ideas bring clarity and hope while the chapter wrap ups index the practical and helpful suggestions.

>Jim "Blinks" Reisinger
>President and Founder
>National Conference on ADD in Adults
>and ADDult Information Exchange Network
>(www.ADDIEN.org)

I like it! This book provides an indexed guide to irritating, self-defeating traits that so many people have. Best of all, it provides practical, easy to apply solutions to these problems in a very organized and accessible format. I plan to recommend this book to my patients and my friends.

>Clifford Corman, M.D.
>Practicing Child Psychiatrist and
>Co-developer of the T.O.V.A.,
>(Test of Variables of Attention)

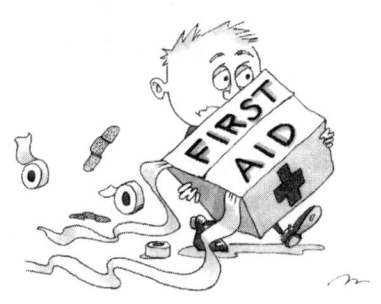